12/05

Brain and Psyche

Brain and Psyche

The Biology of the Unconscious

JONATHAN WINSON

Anchor Press/Doubleday
Garden City, New York
1985

Library of Congress Cataloging in Publication Data

Winson, Jonathan.
  Brain and psyche.

  Includes index.
  1. Subconsciousness—Physiological aspects. 2. Psychoanalysis—Physiological aspects. 3. Brain—Localization of functions. 4. Neuropsychology. I.
Title.
BF315.W56 1984   612'.82   84–2802
ISBN 0-385-19425-0

PERMISSIONS

Illustrations—Flow of visual information on page 19 after drawing in *The Enchanted Loom* by Robert Jastrow, Simon and Schuster, 1981. Alpha rhythm on page 38 adapted from *Mechanics of the Mind* by Colin Blakemore, Cambridge University Press, 1977. Developing neocortex on page 164 from *The Neonatal Development of the Human Cortex* by J. L. Conel, Harvard University Press, 1967. These illustrations have been adapted or reprinted with the kind permission of the publishers.
Quotations—Grateful acknowledgment is made to the following for permission to reprint previously published material: Basic Books, Inc., excerpts from *Collected Papers*, Vol. 1, by Sigmund Freud, copyright 1959 by Basic Books, Inc., and from *The Discovery of the Unconscious* by Henri F. Ellenberger, Copyright 1970 by Henri Ellenberger. Gioia B. Bernheim and Edmund R. Brill: excerpts from the *Interpretation of Dreams* as found in *The Basic Writings of Sigmund Freud*, translated and edited by Dr. A. A. Brill, published by Random House, Inc. (The Modern Library); copyright 1938 (Renewed 1965) by Gioia B. Bernheim and Edmund R. Brill. Princeton University Press, Routledge & Kegan Paul Ltd (London) and The Hogarth Press, excerpts from *The Freud/Jung Letters: The Correspondence Between Sigmund Freud and C. G. Jung*, edited by William McGuire, translated by Ralph Manheim and R.F.C. Hull, Bollingen Series 94. Copyright 1974 by Sigmund Freud Copyrights Ltd. and Erbengenmeinschaft Prof. Dr. C. G. Jung. International Universities Press, Inc., and Sigmund Freud Copyrights Ltd., excerpts from *Psychoanalysis—A General Psychology*, edited by Rudolph M. Loewenstein, Lottie M. Newman, Max Schur, and Albert J. Solnit, copyright 1966 by International Universities Press, Inc. Garland Publishing, Inc., excerpts from *Cat Behavior* by Paul Leyhausen, copyright 1979 by Garland Publishing, Inc.
Illustrations for this book were drawn by Mark Cohen.

To the memory of my parents.

ACKNOWLEDGMENTS:

I want first to express my appreciation to the National Science Foundation, the National Institute of Mental Health, and the Harry Frank Guggenheim Foundation for providing the support that has made my research possible. Larry Squire, Mortimer Mishkin, Torsten Wiesel, Peter Marler, James Ranck, Rosalind Cartwright, and Benjamin Libet, all colleagues in neuroscience or sleep research, have been good enough to review those parts of the book that describe their work. I thank them for their effort and comments. I owe a special debt of gratitude to Patricia Goldman-Rakic and Robin Fox for reviewing the entire manuscript and giving me the benefit of their knowledge. The discussions I had with John Rainer, psychiatrist and training analyst, were invaluable, and I express my appreciation to him. I also gained much from talks with psychoanalyst Arthur Blatt.

Rockefeller University is unique as an institution, as are its graduate students—young scientists in training. Of these students I want to thank most especially Paul Roossin for his precise editorial comments and our many fruitful discussions and to thank Chiye Aoki for her critical reading of the original manuscript. I was fortunate to have Mark Cohen do the illustrations.

I thank my good friends Iris and Bill Willey and Laura and Marvin Mausner for reading the book and giving me the nonscientist's point of view. Lastly I thank my wife, Judy, for her many helpful comments and her constant encouragement and support as I put this book together, and my daughter June for the enthusiasm she conveyed to me throughout the project.

James Raimes, my editor at Doubleday, appraised the manuscript and undertook to help me present it to an audience broader than the scientific community. The book would not have happened without him.

I need only add that I have benefited greatly from the comments I have received, but the responsibility for the views of this book is completely my own.

Contents

Introduction   1

Brain
  One
  MEMORY, PERCEPTION, AND EMOTION   10
  Two
  SLEEP AND DREAMING   35

Psyche
  Three
  THE EARLY DISCOVERIES   62
  Four
  THE INTERPRETATION OF DREAMS   91
  Five
  LATER DEVELOPMENTS   127

Neural Mechanisms
  Six
  CRITICAL PERIOD   162
  Seven
  HIPPOCAMPAL THETA RHYTHM   180
  Eight
  NEURONAL GATING IN THE HIPPOCAMPUS   192

Hypothesis

Nine
HYPOTHESIS   204

Ten
EPILOGUE   241

Notes and References   249

Glossary   283

Index   289

Brain and Psyche

Introduction

And men should know that from nothing else but from the brain come joys, laughter and jests, and sorrows, griefs, despondency and lamentations. And by this, in an especial manner, we acquire wisdom and knowledge, and see and hear and know what are foul and what are fair, what sweet and what unsavory . . . and by the same organ we become mad and delirious and fears and terrors assail us, some by day, and dreams and untimely wanderings, and cares that are not suitable and ignorance of present circumstances, disquietude and unskillfulness. All these things we endure from the brain, when it is not healthy, but is more cold, more moist, or more dry than natural, or when it suffers other preternatural and unusual affliction.

Hippocrates, fifth century B.C.

The remarkably perceptive statement by Hippocrates on the previous page presents what is perhaps the most worthy and challenging goal of science: the understanding of how man's mental life is derived from the physical functioning of his brain. For only with this knowledge can we understand our nature, its origins, and our relationship to all around us.

The problem is very difficult. On the one hand there is the brain, billions of interconnecting neurons, each a highly complicated integrating unit in itself. The brain is truly humbling in its complexity. On the other hand there is man's mental life, ephemeral and ill-defined—described by writers and poets, debated by philosophers, and known in its own version to each person.

About 120 years ago a few insightful physicians began to contribute knowledge to what is currently the field of neuroscience. In England, the neurologist Hughlings Jackson noted that epileptic seizures in his patients sometimes began as a small movement of one part of the body. In a given patient the movement would always be the same. He reasoned that localized irritation of one area of the cerebral cortex, the start of an epileptic attack, caused the motor response, and with this insight he began the study of the cortical control of movement. In Paris, the surgeon Pierre-Paul Broca examined the brains of patients who had, during life, lost the ability to speak and concluded that lesions of a region of the left cerebral cortex were the cause. Broca had localized speech on the left side of the brain. Somewhat later in Spain, the neuroanatomist Santiago Ramon y Cajal, staining neurons in the brains of young animals at early stages of development and meticulously tracing the long slender extensions of the neurons under the microscope, noted that an extension (or axon) of one neuron grew closer to the body of another as the brain developed. He also observed an enlargement at the point where the axon of one neuron finally met the body of another in the mature brain and postulated that neurons do not form a continuous web as was thought at the time, but were individual entities, separated from one another by narrow junctions.

Knowledge in neuroscience has advanced steadily since that time. Neuronal pathways have been traced using ever more sophisticated techniques. The electrical and chemical means by which neurons communicate with one another have been discovered. The discoveries have been remarkable, but each has revealed a new level of complexity. Integrative concepts of how neurons interact so that the brain may perform its function have lagged behind the understanding of the functioning of the individual neuron. A great deal is known about the anatomy and the physiology of the neurons of certain brain structures, for example, and even something of the functions that these individual structures perform. But the neuronal logic of the brain, the way brain structures work in unison to produce psychological function and behavior, is not understood at all.

What of the study of the psyche in its own right, at the level of psychological analysis? There has been one major contribution, made by Sigmund Freud at the beginning of this century. Freud began his career as a neuroscientist. While a medical student at the University of Vienna, he worked in the laboratory of Ernst Brücke, a leading physiologist of his day, pursuing neuroanatomical studies in lower animal species. As a young physician he continued his work in neuroanatomy, specializing in the medulla, a region of the mammalian brain stem. Freud's later history is well known. He became a practicing neurologist, collaborated with Josef Breuer in the treatment of hysteria using the "talking cure," and over a period of several years, developed the psychoanalytic method. The culmination of this process was the publication in 1900 of *The Interpretation of Dreams*, which presented an entire new concept of human personality.

Freud's concept was stunning in its audacity and scope. The answers all seemed to be there. For the first time the mysterious undercurrents of human nature, so long sensed but not understood, were given a cohesive explanation. There was the unconscious—thoughts and wishes of the most primitive kind—repressed, held in check, and kept from conscious awareness by a censor in the mind. Though repressed, these thoughts and wishes had a deep influence on a person's emotional life and behavior—indeed they largely determined personality. This was true in normal individuals. In others, unconscious thoughts were the cause of neurosis, and by uncovering these thoughts via free association during psychoanalysis, one could discover the reason for the neurosis and in many cases cure it. Freud developed these concepts by analyzing his patients' dreams, and as part of his theory he presented another momentous discovery: the meaning of dreams. To Freud, dreams were the expression of primal wishes of the unconscious, which slipped by the mind's censor during sleep when the censor was somewhat relaxed. Freud did not merely state this hypothesis; in *The Interpretation of Dreams* he documented it by meticulously analyzing and classifying many sample dreams.

There followed one of the most ironic chapters of modern intellectual history. Freud's ideas achieved worldwide importance—they came to dominate psychiatry and clinical psychology, and in addition they exerted a profound influence on the culture of Western society. That influence remains, but from the 1950s onward, there has been a decline in acceptance of psychoanalysis as a method of treatment and of Freudian theory as an explanation of the workings of the mind. Psychoanalysis has been supplanted by other means of treating mental disease, and Freudian theory, developed in ever more complex and contradictory layers by Freud in his later years and by his followers, has been widely criticized. As a result, psychoanalysis is today a minority discipline in psychiatry. But through it all, there has been continued recognition of Freud's insight, the accuracy of many of his observations and the pervading feeling that he had revealed a great truth. And no viable alternative theory has been suggested to explain the workings of the human psyche.

There it seems to stand. Neuroscience is slowly unraveling many aspects of brain function, such as the way the sensory world is perceived and remembered and how the brain controls the action of our muscles and bodies. It is working toward, but is still distant from, an understanding of the biology of the psyche. And Freud's theory, somehow still compelling and perhaps containing just out of reach important truths, is in doubt and under challenge to demonstrate its validity.

If a connection could be discovered between the brain in its physical

functioning and the psyche, we would expect a great deal to be clari-
fied. Freud's observations, many of which have been confirmed by psychoanalysts through the years, might be explained on a biological basis.
The understanding of man's nature that we are seeking would be approached.

I suggest in this book that there may be just such a connection. I
believe that certain recent neuroscientific findings provide a link between brain and psyche—a link that begins with an evolutionary
change in the brains of mammals that occurred some 140 million years
ago. This change was retained in the brains of succeeding mammals up
to and including man and, in the brain of man, constitutes the physical
basis of Freud's unconscious. This biological understanding leads to a
new conception of the unconscious as well as of repression and the
meaning of dreams.

This book presents my hypothesis; it traces the connection I see
between brain and psyche. The plan of the book is first to describe
experimental results in two broad areas of neuroscience on which the
hypothesis is based. This is done in the two chapters of the first section
entitled "Brain." The first considers how we perceive and remember
information from the outside world. It begins by tracing a well-known
case history of a man suffering from a severe memory loss. Here the
reader becomes acquainted with some of the mechanisms by which the
brain processes memory. The chapter then goes on to describe how
the brain analyzes and combines the various elements that constitute
the memory of an event—the sights, sounds, and other sensations as
well as any emotions that may be associated with the event. In the
course of the description, the reader is introduced to the hippocampus,
a brain structure intimately associated with memory processing, from
which important clues to the unconscious will later be derived. The
second chapter considers sleep and its evolutionary history. The discovery in the 1950s that dreaming occurs at regular intervals throughout
the night during a distinct phase of sleep is recounted. This discovery
and the story of the evolution of dreaming are two additional clues to
the physical underpinnings of psychological function.

Besides serving the purpose of presenting the physical basis for my
hypothesis, this first section has been designed to give the reader an

overall understanding of the functioning of the brain. Each neuroscientific subject is treated historically. It will be seen how the discoveries were made, and the chapters contain a current account of what is known in each specific area. I have written this description of the brain for the interested layman and it will, I believe, present no difficulty in reading. As an aid, there is a glossary of terms at the back of the book; for those interested in further reading, a section of notes and references lists the original scientific works from which the content of the chapters has been drawn, as well as more detailed comments.

Dreaming is the bridge between brain and psyche. Dreams are associated with an identified physiological process in the brain and are also the prime material Freud used to develop his theories. This bridge is crossed in the second section of the book, entitled "Psyche," which recounts and analyzes the psychological observations and theories of Freud and later psychoanalysts. These sources offer our best clue to the psyche, and my purpose here is to derive from this material the psychological data which may be considered true and for which I hope to find a basis in brain function. Freud's theory of the unconscious and the structure of the psyche were set forth in his book *The Interpretation of Dreams*. The second chapter on Psyche presents the high points of Freud's book. I describe his theories of dreams, repression, and censorship for later comparison with concepts derived from my hypothesis. I begin the section on Psyche with an introductory chapter entitled "Early Discoveries," a short, scientifically oriented biography of Freud up until the time of his publishing *The Interpretation of Dreams*. In addition to describing Freud's early discoveries and how his methods were developed, I have presented the background which gave rise to his particular scientific way of thinking. This becomes important when we later consider his theories. Through an account of his early training, the reader will also become acquainted with the nature of various mental states and aberrations such as hypnosis, multiple personality, and neurosis—states which any comprehensive theory of mental function must explain and which, in a later chapter, I consider in relation to my own hypothesis.

The final chapter on Psyche, "Later Developments," brings the description of psychoanalysis up to date and completes the list of psychological phenomena to be linked with brain function. As with the section on Brain, the section on Psyche serves two purposes. In addition to presenting the psychological observations important for my hypothesis, it will, I believe, give the reader an understanding of the history, content, and current status of psychoanalysis. Here too I list original sources in the Notes and References.

The third section of the book, "Neural Mechanisms," returns to the brain and describes three specific neuroscientific discoveries that constitute three important clues to the relationship between brain and psyche. These are the critical period—relating to the development of the brain early in life—and two neural mechanisms that have been found to operate in the hippocampus: theta rhythm and neuronal gating. As with the earlier section on Brain, the chapter on Critical Period will, I believe, prove to be accessible to lay readers. The chapters which describe neural functioning in the hippocampus are somewhat more complex, but, the details of neural function can be omitted without undue loss. Each of these chapters includes a summary at the end, by which the line of reasoning of the book can be followed.

In the last section of the book, "Hypothesis," all the pieces fit together. I propose a neuroscientific theory to explain Freud's observations. There emerges from this hypothesis a reinterpretation of the meaning of dreams and, from a synthesis of neuroscience and Freud's findings, a view of what the biological origins and makeup of man's nature may be. Man's nature is found to be an unusual product of evolution. It is the joining of a conscious intellect, present only in man, with an unconscious brain mechanism, continually active in every individual, awake and asleep, that has been inherited from our earliest mammalian ancestors. The result is both wondrous and the source of much of man's travail. I discuss these matters as well as how my hypothesis may be tested in the last chapter of the book entitled "Epilogue."

As a neuroscientist, I have found the attempt to understand the relationship between brain and pysche a fascinating endeavor. It has been like trying to solve a grand, scientific detective story, and I hope to share the excitement of this story with the reader in the pages that follow.

Brain

For what is called the physiology of the mind, the development of all kinds of sensations in cases of epilepsy, from the most impersonal (as of sight) to the most personal, the systemic, deserves serious consideration.

Hughlings Jackson
British Medical Journal
February 7, 1874

One

MEMORY, PERCEPTION, AND EMOTION

Memory, Introduction to the Hippocampus

The year was 1953. At the Department of Neurosurgery in the Hartford Hospital in Connecticut, a twenty-nine-year-old man afflicted with epilepsy was being evaluated for surgical treatment. The man, whose initials were H.M., was an intelligent high school graduate who had suffered major seizures since the age of fourteen. The seizures, which occurred without warning, consisted of generalized convulsions accompanied by tongue biting, urinary incontinence, and the loss of consciousness. The attacks had been increasing in frequency and intensity through the years and could not be controlled by anticonvulsant medication. His intellect remained intact, but he was now totally unable to work, and it was hoped that relief might be achieved by means of an admittedly experimental neurosurgical treatment.

This was the era of psychosurgery. The surgical team at Hartford Hospital headed by William Scoville had, over the years preceding 1953, performed several hundred partial prefrontal lobotomies on seriously ill schizophrenic patients. In the then prevalent prefrontal lobotomy procedure, all connecting pathways between the frontal lobes and the underlying brain were severed. Psychotic symptoms were indeed alleviated, but there was a deterioration of personality. Scoville, using his partial lobotomy which cut fewer of the connecting fibers, was attempting to achieve the beneficial effects of total lobotomy on psychosis while avoiding the undesirable effects on personality. He was in fact encouraged by his results.

In a further attempt to improve his procedure, Scoville had gone on from cutting some of the connecting pathways to the frontal lobes to removing a second brain structure, the amygdala, and in some cases a small part of a third, the hippocampus. (These structures lie tucked into the inner wall of the neocortex on each side of the brain.) The amygdala was known to have neural connections to the prefrontal cortex, so Scoville reasoned that still greater benefit might be obtained by destroying this related brain area. The removal of the amygdala and a small part of the hippocampus did not prove to be effective in treating psychosis—but on the positive side it was noted that no additional impairment of mental function occurred as a result of the operation.

Surgery was now considered for the young epileptic patient. The hippocampus was known to be especially prone to seizure activity. Wilder Penfield at the Montreal Neurological Institute had treated epilepsy successfully by removing either the left or right amygdala and hippocampus, though never both. In view of the severity of H.M.'s epilepsy and the apparent lack of impairment of mental function in patients Scoville had operated on, he decided to use the extended surgical procedure and remove H.M.'s amygdala, almost all of his hippocampus, and limited areas of associated neocortex on both sides of the brain. Consequently, on September 1, 1953, Scoville performed this operation.

Following the surgery, H.M.'s epilepsy somewhat improved. (It is currently controlled by medication.) His pleasant preoperative personality was not affected by the operation, nor were his capacity to understand and reason. However, from the time of his surgery to the present, H.M. has suffered from an almost total loss of recent memory. He cannot remember events that have happened only a few moments before. For example, he fails to recognize people he has just met and with whom he may have spent many hours. For years H.M. worked at a state rehabilitation center doing simple manual tasks but during all that period he could never describe his place of work, the nature of his job, or the route along which he was driven every day. Nor can he remember anything about that job today. Having eaten a meal, he will, min-

utes later, not recall the experience and will eat another if it is placed
before him. His mother has described how H.M. will do the same
jigsaw puzzle day after day without any improvement in performance,
as if the puzzle were new each time, and will read the same magazine
over and over again without remembering the content. He has said,
"Every day is alone in itself, whatever enjoyment I've had and whatever
sorrow I've had." In fact, H.M. lives every moment in isolation from
the past.

H.M. has been the subject of intensive study for over twenty-five
years, initially by Brenda Milner of the Montreal Neurological Institute
and later by other neuropsychologists, and a great deal of what is
known about human memory has been learned from him. There are
two striking aspects of his mental deficit that are important in our
present context. The first has to do with new memories as opposed to
old; although H.M. cannot remember new events, he can remember
older ones. The second concerns a certain selectivity of memory loss,
for although he cannot remember new events, he can learn new tasks
that depend on the acquisition of new information.

After his surgery in 1953, H.M. recalled nothing of his hospital stay
immediately preceding the operation. He did not recognize Scoville or
the hospital staff and could not find his way from his room to the
bathroom. This retrograde amnesia has been found to extend some
three years into the past from the time of his operation—that is, to
1950. A favorite uncle of his died in 1950, and each time this event is
mentioned to H.M. he shows renewed surprise and remorse. However,
H.M.'s earlier memories were and continue to be intact. The time
course of his retrograde memory loss was formally tested in 1974. He
was presented with 8×10-inch photographs of eighty-five famous individuals, entertainers, politicians, foreign leaders, Presidents of the
United States, and others who had come to prominence during the
decades from the 1920s through the 1960s, and he was asked to identify these faces. A group of normal men matched to H.M. for age,
background, and intelligence were asked the same questions. H.M.
identified the famous faces of the 1920s, 1930s, and 1940s just as well
as the normal control subjects but he was unable to remember those

who came to prominence in the 1950s and 1960s. The normal men of course remembered the later faces very well.

What tentative conclusions can one draw at this point? If we assume that H.M.'s memory disorder was caused by the bilateral removal of the major part of his hippocampus,* then it would appear that the hippocampus is required for newly occurring events to become available as lasting memories. It appears equally clear that the hippocampus is not necessary for the recollection of older memories. Thus, H.M. recognizes his family and old acquaintances, and he can read, write, and do arithmetic, skills he learned in childhood. However, as we saw, there is a period of about three years just prior to his operation in which older memories have been lost.

Several other cases have come to light which are similar to H.M.'s. In 1957, Scoville and Milner published the first report of the Scoville surgical cases. It appeared that two other patients had undergone removal of the amygdala and the major part of the hippocampus bilaterally several months prior to H.M.'s operation: a woman suffering from manic-depressive psychosis and a paranoid-schizophrenic man. When H.M.'s memory loss was discovered, these patients were tested and found to have the same condition. Their memory impairment had not been noticed before due to their disturbed emotional state. The Scoville patients whose amygdala had been removed but whose hippocampus had not showed some memory problems but not nearly the severe deficits seen when the hippocampus had been removed as well.

H.M.'s syndrome appeared in two of Wilder Penfield's patients who had undergone unilateral amygdaloid and hippocampal removals for epilepsy in the 1940s. In 1975 one of these patients died of unrelated causes, and Penfield performed an autopsy to discover why removing one hippocampus resulted in the memory loss ordinarily associated only with bilateral removal. The autopsy revealed that the hippocampus that had been spared surgically had deteriorated, in all likelihood shortly after birth. Thus the effect of surgery was as if both had been removed. Here, Penfield had taken away only the anterior third of the hippocampus. The syndrome was the same—recent events could not be recalled,

* See Notes and References under page number.

old memories were intact—but the time period preceding the operation in which memories were no longer available was approximately one
year instead of three. The second of Penfield's patients with H.M.'s
syndrome is still alive. In this case, Penfield removed the amygdala and
virtually the entire hippocampus on one side of the brain. Presumably,
here too there is bilateral destruction due to a combination of natural
causes on one side of the brain and surgery on the other. The retrograde amnesia period in this patient is four years.

H.M. is clearly not an isolated case. Bilateral destruction of the
amygdala and hippocampus reduces our view of the world to that of
the moment.

In light of the puzzle presented by the more dramatic aspects of
H.M.'s syndrome, the fact that memories were also lost for a period of
several years prior to the operation was not overly emphasized. But
recent experiments with electroconvulsive therapy in the neuropsychology laboratory of Larry Squire, professor of psychiatry at the University
of California at San Diego, have brought this point into sharper focus.

Electroconvulsive therapy is widely used for severe depression. In its
current form, patients are given an anesthetic and a muscle relaxant.
Electrodes are placed on the skull over the left and right temporal
cortex, and an alternating current is passed between the electrodes for
about half a second. There is no overt convulsion, although there is
electrical seizure activity within the brain. Treatments are usually given
two or three times a week for two to four weeks. The treatment is quite
effective—at times it is the only way to relieve depression. However,
some memory deficit almost always follows its application. The deficit
is reversible; it disappears over a period of seven to nine months following treatment.* Squire and his colleagues have tested patients while the
memory deficit was present and have found that it consists of two
parts. Much like H.M., their patients have difficulty forming new
memories—they cannot retain information beyond a short delay period. This aspect of the memory deficiency recovers considerably
within one month. There is also an amnesia for earlier events, and in
this area Squire's group discovered a most interesting phenomenon.

Squire studied patients undergoing a series of electroconvulsive
shock treatments for depressive illness. He selected twenty-five televi-

sion programs that had appeared for only one season each during the years 1967 through 1974: ten from the 1973–1974 period, seven from the 1970–1972 period, and eight from 1967 and 1968. All had similar Nielsen popularity ratings, so that there was no gross discrepancy in number of times the general public had viewed one program compared to another. Before receiving treatment, the patients were given the name of each program and then were asked to tell all they could remember about the plot, characters, and other details. As might be expected, there was a normal tendency to forget with time. The subjects could remember an average of about twelve facts from the more recent programs and about one fact from programs they had seen seven years before. They then received shock treatments over a period of ten days. One to two hours after the last treatment, the patients were asked to recall once again all they could remember about the same programs. As with H.M., older memories were intact. Thus their recollections of programs approximately seven years old and three to four years old were unchanged by the successive electrical seizures induced by the treatments. However, their ability to recall programs one and two years old was very poor compared to their recollections before treatment. Indeed after treatment, they remembered less about the most recent programs than about programs not seen for three to four years.

In some fashion, older memories, those acquired three or more years before treatment, were being protected from successive electrical seizures while more recent memories were not.

Squire confirmed these findings in other patients and studied the problems carefully. He concluded: "The data strongly support the conclusion that the neural substrate of long-term memory changes for years after learning and that resistance to amnesia develops as a consequence of these changes."

Apparently a slow neural process occurs in the human brain over a period of approximately three years, by which recent events become stabilized as long-term memories. The hippocampus appears to be central to the process, for unless the structure is present and functioning during the three-year period, memories cannot be recalled at a later time. Thus when H.M.'s hippocampus was removed, he could no longer remember the events of the past three years; they were never processed into long-term memory. Also several years of recent memory were erased in Squire's patients who had current passed between their temporal lobes and through their hippocampus, which lies in the path of current flow.*

However once three years have passed, memories are stored in a form that no longer requires the hippocampus for their recall. So H.M. and similar surgical patients retain their older memories although they have no hippocampus. And electroconvulsive therapy does not affect memories that are more than three years old.

The most conservative conclusion these data point to seems to be that the hippocampus plays at least a permissive role in the three-year memory-forming process—that is, the structure makes some contribution, the release of a brain hormone or the like, without which the process cannot occur. The strongest hypothesis would be that the hippocampus is intimately involved in processing memories over a period of several years and that this processing results in long-term memories that are both independent of the hippocampus as far as recall is concerned and resistant to electroconvulsive shocks.

We will return to the hippocampus in this and later chapters, for its role in the functioning of the brain will prove to be an important clue to the biology of the psyche.

I noted earlier that, despite H.M.'s severe memory loss, in many respects his mental functioning is normal. His personality is relatively unchanged. He can read, write, and do arithmetic. All of this is understandable in view of his retention of the memories of older events and experiences.* But there was one unusual finding. Neuropsychologists testing him found that his perception, his ability to reason abstractly, and his ability to learn new tasks were unaffected by removal of his hippocampus, providing the tasks depended on learning rules of procedure—that is, what step or move follows what—rather than the recollection of events unconnected to one another by such rules.

An example of H.M.'s perceptual skills was his performance on the Mooney test. Here the subjects are shown a chaotic black and white pattern in which a face with incomplete boundaries is hidden. They must find the face in the pattern and give the sex and approximate age of the person they see. H.M. responded quickly and accurately to forty-four such test patterns presented in succession, surpassing the performance of age-matched control subjects. But when shown twelve photographs of faces, then distracted for ninety seconds and asked to select these faces from twenty-five faces, he could not remember the twelve faces at all. His performance was random.

H.M. readily learned a task involving both perceptual and motor skills. Brenda Milner tested him over a three-day period on his ability to guide a pencil between two boundary lines, when he could see the movement of his own hand only in a mirror. Each day he was unaware that he had been tested the day before. Yet his learning curve was normal—he began each new session at the advanced level he had reached on the previous day.

Within the last several years, H.M. has been asked to, and has successfully solved, increasingly sophisticated puzzles. An example is the puzzle of the Tower of Hanoi. Five disks of successively smaller size, with holes in their centers, are placed on a peg in order of size, the smallest on top. There are two other pegs in a row, without disks. The task is to transfer the disks to the most distant peg so that they are in the same size order, the smallest on top. Transfers can be made one disk at a time to or from any peg, but a larger disk may never be placed over a smaller one. H.M. arrived at a solution to this rather complex problem by trial and error over a period of daily sessions in a manner similar to normal control subjects, yet for any given trial he believed he was seeing the puzzle for the very first time.

What is the basis for this unusual split of function between memory of events and procedural memory? How is the three-year period of memory consolidation to be explained? These questions are currently being studied in a number of neuroscientific laboratories. It is believed that the answers will ultimately be found in an understanding of neuroanatomy and neurophysiology. In the remaining part of this chapter I will present some idea of what is known of the anatomy and function of brain structures most intimately involved with the phenomena I have been describing. I will pay special attention to the hippocampus as one of our links to psychological function.

Perception

Perhaps the best way to begin is to consider the way the brain processes a sensory input such as vision—how we "see" a visual scene. The lens of the eye first focuses a visual scene onto the retina, where it impinges on photosensitive receptor cells—over 100 million such cells in the retina of each eye. Information is processed within the retina itself, culminating in the activation of neurons called ganglion cells (a neuron is a cell in the nervous system specialized for the transmission of information). Approximately 1 million ganglion cells carry the output of the retina to the first level of processing within the brain itself— a group of neurons in the thalamus called the lateral geniculate nucleus. The thalamus is a brain structure lying beneath the neocortex, intimately connected with it both anatomically and functionally. For each of the senses—vision, hearing, touch, and taste—there is a relay in the thalamus before information is passed to the neocortex. (The organization of the sense of smell is a bit different.) From the thalamus, the next receiving area in the brain for visual information is in the neocortex proper, specifically an area in its back portion called primary visual or striate cortex.

Like most neurons, the ganglion cell transmits its information by means of an electrical pulse (an action potential), which travels down its output fiber (the axon). An action potential is triggered in the cell body when inputs to the cell from other neurons reach a sufficient level of intensity. These input signals are received by a neuron on thin fibrous extensions of the cell called dendrites as well as on the cell body itself. A neuron is generally bombarded by constantly changing inputs at what may be thousands of locations on its dendrites and body, some of these inputs tending to excite the cell toward firing an action potential and others tending to inhibit firing. Each neuron acts as a complex biological integrating machine, firing one or more action potentials along its axon (and thus transmitting its message to one or more target

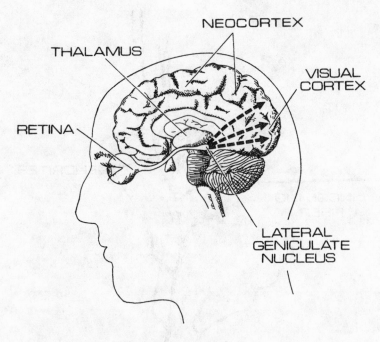

NEOCORTEX

THALAMUS

VISUAL
CORTEX

RETINA

LATERAL
GENICULATE
NUCLEUS

ILLUSTRATION 1

Visual processing begins in the retina of the eye, which contains the ganglion cells. The axons of the ganglion cells carry the signals to the lateral geniculate nucleus, part of the thalamus, which is the first relay station in the brain for analyzing visual images. The signals are then sent to the primary visual cortex. The two sides of the brain work in coordination to produce the visual image. The part of the visual scene to the left of where the eyes are directed is processed by the right side of the brain, while images in the right visual field are processed on the left side. The split visual fields are then joined to re-create the original image.

neurons), depending on the timing of its many inputs and on the particular way the neuron combines its incoming signals.

The actual transmission of a neuron to the dendrite or cell body of a target neuron is accomplished chemically. The far end of the axon lies very close to the dendrite or cell body of the target neuron but does not actually touch it. The junction between the axon and the target cell is called the synapse, and the very narrow channel separating the end of

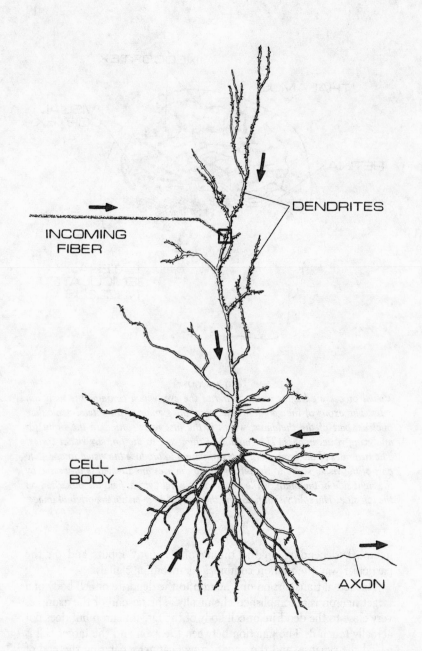

INCOMING
FIBER

DENDRITES

CELL
BODY

AXON

ILLUSTRATION 2

Illustrated is a neuron of the visual cortex, a pyramidal cell, so named because of the shape of its cell body, which resembles a pyramid. There is a complex arborization of dendrites (fibrous extensions of the cell which receive inputs from other neurons), a cell body and a single output fiber or axon, which transmits signals in the form of action potentials from the cell to other neurons. (The direction of the flow of information, from the dendrites through the cell body and out through the axon, is shown by arrows.) Although the cell has but a single axon, this axon may branch later on in its path and activate many target neurons. The cell itself is a complex neural machine integrating inputs and firing action potentials according to its own inbuilt logic. Neurons may take many forms, but almost all consist of the same three basic elements—dendrites, cell body, and axon. An incoming fiber from another neuron is shown transmitting its signal to a dendrite. The junction point of the incoming fiber and dendrite, surrounded by a box, is shown enlarged in the illustration on the next page.

the transmitting axon from the receiving dendrite or cell body is called the synaptic cleft. When an action potential reaches the synapse at the end of the axon, it releases a chemical substance, a neurotransmitter, into the synaptic cleft. The neurotransmitter acts locally upon the receiving cell where, for a few thousandths of a second, it changes the permeability of the cell wall or membrane to chemical ions, which are present in the extracellular fluid in and around the synaptic cleft. The consequent flow of these ions through the cell wall excites or inhibits the target cell.

Nature's provision of a chemical link at the synapse is a most fortunate circumstance. It makes possible medical intervention into brain function, since drugs taken orally and consequently carried in the bloodstream can reach the synapse and influence the action of neurotransmitters. We shall see later how drugs acting on particular neurotransmitters have dramatically altered the treatment of mental disease.

Returning to our analysis of vision, let us consider the information that the brain will ultimately extract from a visual scene. The scene may include a tree, a cloud, a building, an automobile, an animal, or a person. Each of these is characterized by a distinct shape, color or colors, texture, and depth. We recognize each whether it is near or far and can judge its relative distance from us. If the object is moving, we continue to recognize it and can judge its direction and speed. How does the brain perform this task?

David Hubel and Torsten Wiesel at Harvard University studied visual processing at the level of the primary visual cortex in cats and monkeys, and their work has made aspects of this processing clear. The retina does not treat the visual scene as a whole; it analyzes the scene in small, overlapping circular patches. It is as if a photograph were cov-

ILLUSTRATION 3

The synapse is the junction point at which a neuron transmits its signal to another target neuron. The axon of the signaling neuron ends in a knobby tip, which contains vesicles filled with neurotransmitter. The knobby end of the axon lies very close to the membrane (postsynaptic membrane) of a dendrite or the cell body of the target neuron, but does not actually touch it. A narrow channel or synaptic cleft separates the two. The arrival of an action potential at the axon tip causes neurotransmitter to be released into the synaptic cleft, where it acts to open channels in the postsynaptic membrane. The flow of ions (substances such as sodium and potassium dissolved in the extracellular fluid surrounding the synapse) through these open channels provides an input, which either excites the target cell to fire an action potential or inhibits firing.

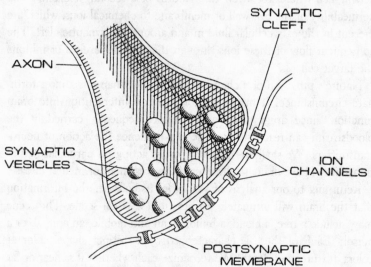

ered by overlapping circles.* The retina transmits the visual scene from these small circular patches all at one time. This is parallel processing. In contrast, a television camera viewing the scene would scan it in successive horizontal sweeps, from top to bottom, thus processing the image sequentially.

When the information about the scene reaches the lateral geniculate nucleus, the brain continues to analyze the visual scene in terms of the patterns of reflected light that fall upon the small circular areas of the visual field. In cats or monkeys it is possible to monitor the firing of action potentials in one individual neuron in the lateral geniculate nucleus. In a darkened room, the animal's eyes are focused on a screen on which is projected a spot of light. Each neuron will respond to the spot of light only when it is within a particular small circular area of the screen, its visual field. The cell fires most rapidly when the spot of light is focused at the center of this small area.*

The ultimate scheme of processing by which the brain analyzes the visual world is suggested when one studies what happens in the primary visual cortex. Here two types of information begin to be extracted. There are neurons that respond to lines projected on the screen rather than to spots. Furthermore, different neurons respond to different slants of lines with respect to the vertical. It would appear that spot detectors of the retina and lateral geniculate nucleus have combined their information; they have lined up their spots in a row to become line detectors, and indeed line detectors sensitive to the particular orientation or slant of a line. Presumably, this is the first stage by which the form or shape of objects will finally be identified. Also, side-by-side in the primary visual cortex are neurons that respond to the same orientation of a line as seen in the same part of the visual field by either eye. However, one neuron will respond more strongly to an input from the left eye, and its neighbor will respond more strongly to an input from the right eye. This information about the same part of the visual scene as seen by either eye will be used to organize depth perception. All the individual receptive fields of the cortical neurons overlap at their edges to form a full representation of the visual scene in the primary visual cortex. But now the line orientation and depth information at each place in the scene is available for further processing.

Surrounding the primary visual cortex and receiving inputs from it are other cortical areas in which there are many separate representations of the visual field. At least thirteen representations have been found in the owl monkey. Each of these areas apparently performs a separate function of feature extraction in the analysis of the visual scene—further steps in the perception of form, as well as the detection of color, texture, depth, and motion. Neurons have been found in these regions that are specifically sensitive to color, texture, and depth. But perhaps the most interesting question concerns the analysis of shape or form. Are shape detectors built out of detectors of lines of different orientations and length, much as line detectors are thought to be built from the combined inputs of spot detectors? The neural scheme for this process is unknown, but the anatomical area in which it culminates may be the inferotemporal cortex. Much as the primary visual cortex sends inputs to adjacent feature detection areas, so these areas send

ILLUSTRATION 4

The human neocortex as seen from the left side. The neocortex is a large sheet of tissue about 1/10 inch thick. The infolded convolutions that are seen are due to the squeezing together and hence the folding of the sheet to fit within the confines of the skull. The upper figure shows the regions in which the neocortex processes sensory information. At the back of the brain is the primary visual cortex, where the processing of visual images begins; toward the front and lower portion of the brain is the inferotemporal cortex, part of the temporal lobe. Neocortical areas with various feature detectors lie between the two. Visual information is believed to be processed sequentially from the primary visual to the inferotemporal cortex as indicated by the arrows (after Mortimer Mishkin). Shown also are the areas that analyze hearing and touch. Taste and smell are processed by parts of the neocortex not visible from the outside of the brain.

Regions of the neocortex that deal with other functions are shown in the lower figure. At the front of the brain is the prefrontal cortex, the area undercut during prefrontal lobotomy. The function of the prefrontal cortex is discussed in Chapter 2. Next to it is the region that governs movement. The parietal cortex is an area in which sensory inputs are integrated; it is concerned at least in part with spatial relations among parts of the body and between the body and objects of the outside world. A number of functions are controlled primarily by one neocortical hemisphere, the left or the right. Language is centered in the left hemisphere as shown; spatial imagery is centered in the right.

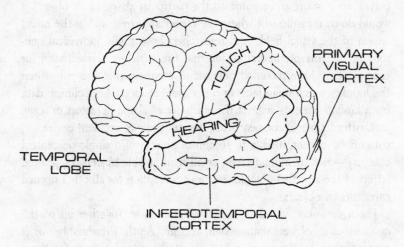

TOUCH

PRIMARY
VISUAL
CORTEX

HEARING

TEMPORAL
LOBE

INFEROTEMPORAL
CORTEX

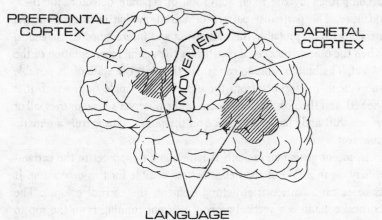

PREFRONTAL
CORTEX

MOVEMENT

PARIETAL
CORTEX

LANGUAGE

inputs to the inferotemporal region. Neurons here respond to visual stimuli but not to other sensory inputs such as sound or touch. The receptive fields here are very large. If a neuron in the inferotemporal cortex were to fire in response to the particular shape of an object, it would do so regardless of where the object appeared within the broad region of the visual field. And researchers have found individual neurons in the inferotemporal cortex that fire with great selectivity; for example they have recorded neurons in monkeys that fire only when the monkey sees human faces or other monkey faces. Also, clinical data from human patients suggest the existence of shape detectors of some sort. After lesions of the neocortex, due generally to accident or disease, patients have been unable to recognize objects of a single perceptual category—such as human faces, small manipulable objects, or printed letters of the alphabet—while retaining perception for all other normal categories of objects.

For a complete visual image, the brain draws together all of the qualities of an object: shape, color, texture, depth. Presumably this is accomplished by the rapid activation of separate detectors for these qualities. The particular pattern of activation that occurs within the neocortex (and probably the underlying and interconnected thalamus) when the object is observed constitutes the neural representation of the object. The brain is able to categorize the object in spite of its possible movement, its distance from the observer, the angle from which it is viewed, and the possible movement of the observer's head or eyes, all of which shift and change the image on the retina. This is truly a remarkable feat.

In recent years neuroscientists have come to appreciate the extraordinary organization of the neocortex responsible for this processing. It is based on a particular structural element, the cortical column. The cortical column is a vertical array of neurons running from the top to the bottom surface of the neocortex, a distance of about one tenth of an inch. (The basic thin neocortical sheet is folded on itself within the skull, accordionlike, to form convolutions as is shown in the figures on pages 19 and 25.)

The diameter of each column is approximately one to two thousandths of an inch, and each contains about 110 neurons in all parts of the neocortex except in the primary visual cortex, where it contains a little more than twice that number. The column is an input-output device which, in the sensory systems, performs the function of local feature extraction. For example, in the visual system we have been discussing, an individual column in the primary visual cortex may contain neurons that respond most strongly to a visual stimulus at one particular part of the visual field as seen by one eye and may extract a single feature, say lines slanted 10 degrees to the right of the vertical. Next to it are successive columns that extract lines of successively greater inclinations to the vertical so that within a patch of visual cortex of about 15 thousandths of an inch, lines of any orientation at that point in the visual field would be detected.*

The cortical column was first discovered in 1957 by Vernon Mountcastle of Johns Hopkins University, who was working in the area of the neocortex that analyzes body sensations such as touch. Mountcastle found that neurons in a given column responded to sensations from a particular point of the body; further, these neurons were sensitive to only a single body sensation such as deep pressure, light pressure, or sensations from body joints. The generality of the column in sensory processing was strongly reinforced by the findings of Hubel and Wiesel in the visual system I have just described. Columnar processing has also been found in hearing; columns act to detect frequency of sound, the ear in which the sound is heard, and even the time lag between the reception of sound by one ear and the other (which allows the hearer to localize the source of the sound in space). Neocortical areas responsible for movement and higher associational processes were also found to be organized into columns. Indeed, it appears the entire neocortex consists of a vast array of interconnected columns: an estimated 600 million constituting 50 billion neurons in all.

We have not yet reached the hippocampus in our description. The prodigious apparatus we have described is neocortical, and it should therefore not be surprising that H.M., neocortex and lower brain centers intact, should retain his perceptual abilities. Asked to discern a face in the chaotic background, his feature detectors perform normally. Long before his surgery, H.M. had learned how to perceive a face. This older perceptual ability was not disturbed by the removal of his hippocampus and amygdala, so he can recognize a face and categorize it. Asked to do mirror drawing, the pattern he is asked to draw in reversed fashion is in front of him to be perceived directly, without the use of memory. To sum up, H.M.'s motor skills and his ability to reason or follow rules are within the capacity of his neocortex and lower brain centers and so he can learn to perform perceptual tasks.*

We finally turn to the hippocampus and amygdala. These structures are tucked under the inner wall of the temporal lobe of the neocortex. I have described the flow and sequential analysis of the visual sensory information from the primary visual cortex to the inferotemporal cortex. As conceived by Mortimer Mishkin of the National Institute of Mental Health, whose research has been important in clarifying neural

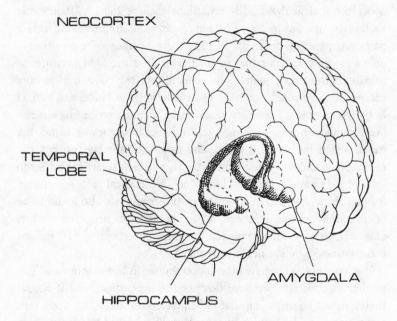

ILLUSTRATION 5
The hippocampus is a bilateral, elongated, sausagelike structure tucked into the inner wall of the temporal cortex. The amygdala is a brain nucleus or assembly of cells lying immediately in front of it.

processing of this nature, information in other senses such as hearing and possibly touch are also processed with increasing refinement as one proceeds to other (nonvisual) parts of the temporal lobe. Just as the activation of the various visual feature extractors serves to represent the visual world in the brain at a given moment, so the simultaneous activation of all sensory feature detectors represents the entire sensory world at that moment. Mishkin finds that all sensory systems send inputs to the amygdala, each sensory system to a separate part of that structure. The function of the amygdala is not clearly understood, but based on indirect evidence I will describe later, one may say that it is concerned with emotion, and that particular sensory inputs may be associated with a particular emotional tone in the amygdala and in other brain structures to which it sends its output. This information is ultimately transmitted to the hippocampus.

All of the neocortical sensory systems that give rise to separate inputs to the amygdala also send inputs to a neocortical area called the entorhinal cortex. Here the sensory inputs converge, and a major input is sent to the hippocampus. The net result of all the processing of information that I have described is this: If we consider an event as made up of a confluence of sensory inputs that occurs over a short period of time, then the highest order of perceptual abstraction of these sensory inputs together with an emotional association are presented to the hippocampus for processing. And as we have learned from H.M., this processing is necessary for the event to enter memory.*

Emotion

To conclude this chapter, I turn to the relationship of the hippocampus to a group of structures collectively called the limbic system. It is believed that within the limbic system, a series of brain processes occurs by which perception and memory affect thought, feeling, and behavior.

The hippocampus is a pivotal component of the limbic system. The term "limbic" was originally an anatomical designation given by Pierre-

Paul Broca in 1876 to a ring of brain tissue containing the hippocampus, amygdala, and other structures that formed a border (limbus) around a ventricle or fluid-filled cavity in the center of the brain, the foramen of Monro. The brain, excluding the brain stem, may be conceived of as two concentric shells surrounding this central ventricle. The inner shell contains the hippocampus, amygdala, and other related structures. This is the limbic lobe. The second and outer shell, which surrounds the limbic lobe, is the neocortex. The term "limbic system" was introduced much more recently, in 1952 by Paul McLean, head of the Laboratory of Brain Evolution and Behavior of the National Institutes of Health, to designate a series of structures of the limbic lobe as well as others closely related anatomically, which were believed to serve a common function related to emotion.

Each component of the limbic system is a highly organized processing unit whose internal mechanisms are, at best, poorly understood. The components bear these names: hippocampus, amygdala, septum, mammillary bodies, anterior thalamic nuclei, and cingulate cortex. Brain structures were often named by early anatomists on the basis of their external shape. Thus the hippocampus was thought to resemble the small, marine sea horse (and so was called hippocampus, the Greek word for sea horse), amygdala means almond, and the mammillary bodies are a twin pair of breast-shaped structures.

The structures of the limbic system are interconnected in a complex series of circuits. I pointed out earlier in this chapter that sensory information, assembled in ever more complete form by processing in successive neocortical stages, finally reaches the hippocampus and constitutes its major input. A large and important circuit then connects the hippocampus to several of the other limbic structures, and from these, connections reach the remaining limbic system components. This pattern of connectivity makes one point clear. The hippocampus is the gateway from the neocortex to the rest of the limbic system. Additionally, the hippocampus, as well as each of the other limbic structures, receives important inputs from the brain stem, a subject which we will return to in a later chapter. (The limbic system is illustrated on page 33.)

In the face of this anatomic complexity, what have neuroscientists been able to learn about limbic system function? The limbic system appears to act as a central core information processing system in the brain that is interposed between sensory input and motor output (movement of the body). The structures within it do not receive any direct sensory input; rather they deal with highly organized information derived from events, memories of events, and emotions associated with those events. Nor do the structures directly affect motor function, although behavior, on the level of the choice of behavior rather than detailed fine movement, is certainly strongly influenced by limbic system processing.

This concept of limbic system function has been derived both from its neuroanatomy and from observing behaviors in humans and animals after accidental or experimental destruction of particular limbic structures. The association of the limbic system with emotion was first suggested in 1937 by James Papez, a neuroanatomist. He considered the known connections among structures of the limbic system as well as published reports of emotional symptoms resulting from lesions of these structures in humans and monkeys, and wrote in a now classic paper entitled "A Proposed Mechanism of Emotion":

> It is proposed that the hypothalamus [mammillary body], the anterior thalamic nuclei, the gyrus cinguli [cingulate gyrus], and the hippocampus and their connections constitute a harmonious mechanism which may elaborate the functions of the central emotion, as well as participate in emotional expression.

In this article, Papez also presented a mechanism by which emotion was linked to the rest of consciousness, a mechanism based on the path of information flow through the components of the limbic system.*

Papez's main contribution was his suggestion that a specific anatomical circuit underlay emotional feeling and thought. His general views regarding emotion have been largely sustained, but not his specific analysis of the flow of information within the limbic system. This is now being worked out more in accordance with the chain of information processing from neocortex to hippocampus and amygdala (described earlier in this chapter) and from there to other components of the system.

In 1939, two years after Papez's paper appeared, Heinrich Klüver and Paul Bucy at the University of Chicago reported the results of experiments in monkeys that reinforced Papez's idea. They made very large brain lesions in their animals, removing the amygdala, the hippocampus, and the temporal lobes of the neocortex on both sides of the brain. These lesions resulted in drastic emotional symptoms—the so-called Klüver-Bucy syndrome. The monkeys used were wild, and typically such animals, when turned loose in a room with an experimenter, run to find a secure place away from the experimenter or crouch and remain still and then suddenly dash away. After the lesions, these animals approached any object without hesitation: the experimenter, a large snake, even a monkey that had previously attacked them. In addition they exhibited bizarre hypersexuality—in males, hours of copulation, masturbation, or homosexual behavior. They also indiscriminately put both edible and inedible objects in their mouths.

Many lesion experiments of a more refined nature as well as experiments in which brain areas have been stimulated electrically and consequent behavior noted have sustained the impression that the limbic system—and in particular the amygdala—is related to emotion. In-

ILLUSTRATION 6

The limbic system is made up of a series of interconnected structures surrounding a central fluid-filled ventricle of the forebrain and forming an inner border of the cerebral cortex. The structures include the hippocampus, amygdala, septum, anterior thalamic nuclei, mammillary bodies, and cingulate cortex. The fornix is a long fiber bundle joining the hippocampus to the mammillary bodies. The limbic system is shown in place in the brain in the upper figure and is shown in an enlarged view below. Pictured also are the corpus callosum, a fiber tract joining right and left neocortex, the cerebellum, a structure involved in modulating movement, and the brain stem. The limbic system is neither directly sensory nor motor but constitutes a central core processing system of the brain that deals with information derived from events, memories of events, and emotional associations to these events. This processing is essential if experience is to guide future behavior.

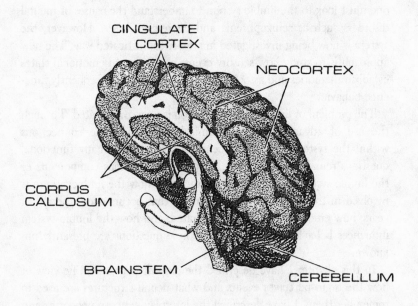

CINGULATE
CORTEX

NEOCORTEX

CORPUS
CALLOSUM

BRAINSTEM

CEREBELLUM

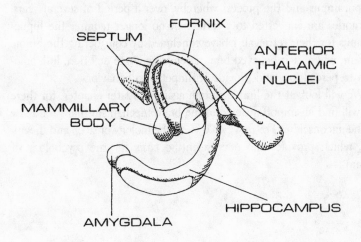

SEPTUM

FORNIX

ANTERIOR
THALAMIC
NUCLEI

MAMMILLARY
BODY

AMYGDALA

HIPPOCAMPUS

deed, neuroscientists and biologically oriented psychiatrists believe that one must look to the limbic system to understand the causes of mental disorders such as schizophrenia and depressive illness. However, the system is now being investigated in a more sophisticated way. The new approach is to study how sensory events coupled with emotional states establish memories and associations, and how these consequently influence behavior.

The problem of limbic system function is very complicated. Through the use of advanced neuroanatomical techniques, the connections within the system are rapidly being unraveled. But many functional questions remain, such as the extent to which various components of the limbic system are necessary for memory; how the limbic system is involved in the consolidation of memory that occurs over a period of years; how emotional states are generated; and how the limbic system influences behavior. The answers to these questions are presently unknown.

In this chapter I have described the current neuroscientific view of how the brain perceives events and what neural structures are used to remember them. I have described the interplay between neocortex and hippocampus and the process whereby, over a period of several years, memories are converted to a form that no longer requires the hippocampus for their retrieval. I have concluded by considering the limbic system, where it is believed brain circuits generate emotion, link emotion to perception, and provide an impetus to behavior.

We will look at the limbic system again in a later chapter, for there we will find an important clue to the brain mechanism that Freud saw as the unconscious. For now, we turn to the biology of sleep and dreaming, which provides the neuroscientific basis for the psychology of dreams.

Two

SLEEP AND DREAMING

Nathaniel Kleitman, professor of physiology at the University of Chicago, had long been interested in the study of sleep. He was one of a small group of investigators in the laboratories around the world who, during the 1930s and 1940s, were attempting to understand this elusive state. They began with the common knowledge of the time that sleep was the regularly occurring other state of consciousness which seemed to be required for the periodic restitution of bodily energy or reserves. Dreaming occurred during sleep. Its frequency of occurrence and duration were unknown.

Applying the scientific tools then available, Kleitman and the other scientists measured various physiological indices such as temperature, heart rate, respiratory rate, and blood pressure during the waking-sleeping cycle. Body movement was also monitored. Most important for the course of future research, the electroencephalographic (EEG) signals generated by the neocortex were recorded during sleep. More will be said about the EEG later, but for now it should be mentioned that in the early 1930s it was found possible to record, from the surface of the skull, the electrical activity of the neocortical neurons lying beneath it, and sleep researchers took these recordings in a number of subjects throughout a night's sleep.

In Kleitman's laboratory, body temperature was found to vary cyclically over a twenty-four-hour period. It was lowest at midnight and highest at noon. This twenty-four-hour temperature variation developed gradually over the first year of an infant's life as did the sleep-wakefulness cycle. Heart rate was found to be lower during sleep than during the waking state. Blood pressure was also somewhat depressed during sleep. Reports on respiratory rate from various laboratories were contradictory—some measured an increase and some a decrease during sleep. In all of these experiments, sleep was considered to be a single physiological state present throughout the night, and the physiological measures reported were average values taken for an entire night's sleep. As we shall see, sleep is not a single physiological state, but consists of several. Meaningful changes in the physiological measures did indeed occur during particular phases of sleep, but were not detected due to the averaging procedure.

Kleitman attempted a number of manipulations of sleep, probing for its mechanisms and functions. Two experiments give the flavor of his research. First, Kleitman tried to alter the twenty-four-hour temperature cycle he had discovered. He had a subject sleep four hours in every twelve instead of the normal eight-hour period once a night, hoping that he might entrain the temperature cycle to the twelve-hour sleep cycle. However the twenty-four-hour temperature cycle was maintained. He then tried a forty-eight-hour sleep cycle. He and an associate slept for only one night out of two over a ten-day period. Again the twenty-four-hour temperature cycle persisted. It seemed there was an internal biological clock maintaining a twenty-four-hour temperature cycle independent of sleep.

Finally in 1938, in a more elaborate experiment which received some publicity at the time, Kleitman and another associate tested whether the twenty-four-hour temperature cycle could be modified if the sleep-waking cycle were shifted only moderately from the normal twenty-four hours. They spent thirty-four days in a chamber in Mammoth Cave, Kentucky, living on a twenty-eight-hour schedule. Light was on for nineteen hours a day and off for nine hours, during which the subjects slept. It was found that one man's temperature cycle did shift smoothly into a twenty-eight-hour rhythm while the other man's stubbornly maintained a twenty-four-hour rhythm despite its lack of synchrony with the lighting and sleeping cycle. It appeared that the rhythm of the biological clock governing temperature control could be changed to a small extent in some individuals but not in others. This type of research which deals with circadian (about twenty-four hours) variations of physiological function continues to be an important branch of sleep research today, dealing with, among other questions, the physiological basis of jet lag.

In a second experiment, Kleitman used a classic approach: to discover the function of an entity, remove it, and observe the consequences. Thirty-five students volunteered to stay awake for a period of approximately sixty hours. A rotating series of watchers observed each subject and kept him awake for approximately eighty hours, four days and three nights. During the first night the students were able to stay awake, reading or doing laboratory work, without too much attention from the watchers. They became drowsy but could shake it off. During the second night their desire for sleep was almost overpowering. They often saw double. On the third day they could no longer write; the attempt led to unintelligible scribbling, or the students dropped their pencils. If they attempted to count to 15 or 20 they would lose track of the numbers and doze off.

Subjects became irascible and somewhat irrational. A student would make a remark that was clearly not appropriate to the situation. When questioned about it, he would say that he was talking to the watcher on a topic which had, in reality, never been mentioned. The students remained in this state through the third night and the fourth day of sleeplessness, but then after a long night's sleep they fully recovered. Throughout the period of sleep deprivation, their vital bodily functions were found to be normal. The only noteworthy physiological change was a decrease in the threshold to pain. Most of the effects that did occur seemed to be an intensification of the reactions that are commonly experienced with a less severe loss of sleep.

These experiments are examples of hundreds that were performed on humans and animals between 1930 and 1950. Although much information was gathered, it all appeared somehow to be peripheral. An understanding of sleep remained elusive.

It was hoped that the EEG would provide a clue. Hans Berger, a German psychiatrist, made the initial discovery. In a series of papers published between 1929 and 1933 he reported an electrical effect which could be detected in human subjects by electrodes applied to the scalp. It consisted of a rhythmic oscillation of electrical potential with a frequency of about 10 per second, which appeared when the subject lay quietly with his eyes closed. The rhythmic potential disappeared when the subject opened his eyes to observe a visual scene. Berger was intrigued by this effect (called the Berger rhythm by early workers, and the alpha rhythm at a later time). He considered it a reflection of mental events and believed the *Elektroenkephalogramm* that recorded it might provide a link between brain function and psychology.

Scientists at the time were dubious. Berger's equipment was crude; the alpha rhythm might be an artifact—that is, something artificially produced by the test equipment rather than a naturally occurring phenomenon. Workers doubted that such uniform activity could occur in the brain of a conscious subject. But in 1934 at the prestigious neurophysiological laboratory in Cambridge, England, Edgar Adrian and colleagues repeated Berger's experiments, confirmed the basic result, and provided additional findings. Berger thought that the entire neocortex was involved in generating the alpha rhythm, since he had detected it from all parts of the scalp. Adrian demonstrated that the rhythm originated in the primary visual cortex at the back of the brain. The fact that the alpha rhythm could be recorded all over the scalp was due to the method of recording. The skull, which has a high electrical

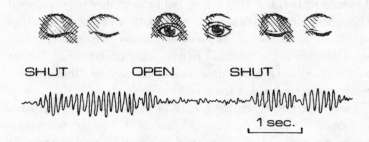

SHUT   OPEN   SHUT

|⎯⎯ 1 sec. ⎯⎯|

ILLUSTRATION 7

Hans Berger, a German psychiatrist, discovered the alpha rhythm in the early 1930s. Edgar Adrian confirmed Berger's discovery of the alpha rhythm and demonstrated that it came from the primary visual cortex. This is the record of alpha rhythm recorded from the scalp of Adrian himself. The 10 per second rhythm appeared when he lay awake with his eyes closed. It disappeared when he opened his eyes and reappeared when he shut them again.

resistance, was interposed between the scalp electrode and the generating neurons in the neocortex. Recording through this resistance was equivalent to recording without the resistance but from a much greater distance from the surface of the cortex. Thus, the EEG reflected the average electrical activity of neurons within a broad cortical region. An electrode would tend to receive a stronger signal from an area of neocortex lying directly beneath it, but it would also detect a prominent rhythm such as the alpha rhythm generated anywhere in the cortex.

What was the alpha rhythm? Presumably it reflected the synchronous, periodic activation of large numbers of visual cortex neurons at a rate of 10 times per second. In contrast, when a subject opened his eyes and focused on a visual scene, the neurons of the various regions of his visual cortex could be expected to fire in some complex, nonsynchronous fashion as the neurons became engaged in the analysis of the features of the scene. There would be no periodic rise and fall of electrical activity. The electrical signal recorded by the EEG would represent the average electrical activity of many cells firing in different patterns, and one would expect a low-level, random signal. This is just the type of signal seen when a subject, in whom alpha rhythm is being recorded, opens his eyes. An analogy may be drawn between the EEG and the sound detected by a sensitive microphone suspended over a large assemblage of people conversing with one another. No individual conversation would be discerned but the general noise level would be detected. This is equivalent to the "eyes open" EEG. Should the assemblage all fall silent or raise their voices at once, the effect would be detected by the microphone—an effect like the alpha rhythm.

Despite considerable research at the time, scientists could not discover the significance or the function of the alpha rhythm—nor is it known today. Speculation at the time centered upon some sort of internal scanning mechanism operating in the visual cortex under the condition of resting with closed eyes, such as occurs preceding sleep, but there has been no evidence to support this idea.

In the light of this background, it was natural for investigators to use the EEG in the study of sleep. By the mid 1930s the first results were being reported. As a subject drifted into sleep, the alpha rhythm gave way to a bewildering array of other EEG patterns. There were periods during sleep when the EEG signal was similar to the alert waking state. Then there were periods when so-called spindles at 14 per second lasting 1/2 to 1 second appeared, and periods when "random" potentials at 2 to 3 per second filled the EEG record. The different types of EEG pattern seemed to follow one another in cycles through the night. An important conclusion was drawn—one could no longer think of sleep as a single continuous state. There was a series of shifts from one sleep state to another.

One group of investigators reported that dreams were associated with a particular EEG state, the state in which the EEG pattern was low-level and random. Two subjects had awakened from this state and had reported dreams. Other researchers disagreed. An experiment in which Kleitman had participated found that dreams occurred throughout sleep. Another laboratory concluded that dreams could occur in association with any EEG pattern but were more likely to occur during particular patterns, one of which was the low-level random signal. The data were confusing—there was no apparent order in the EEG signals. And yet within these data there lie evidence of a basic biological mechanism.

The pivotal study came in 1951. Kleitman was to say later that his laboratory "stumbled" into it. Eugene Aserinsky, a graduate student, and Kleitman were preparing for a series of experiments in which they would study the body movements of infants one to seven months old during sleep. The infants would be observed in their cribs during daytime sleep and their periodic movements recorded by a device attached to the spring of each crib. They were known to show a 50–60 minute cycle of movement during sleep, and studying this motility cycle was one of Kleitman's ongoing interests. For this experiment a new variable was going to be observed. It had been noted that when infants stirred periodically, their eyes moved under closed lids. Aserinsky and Kleitman were going to note carefully and record these eye movements.

These movements turned out to be a more consistent indicator of the motility cycle than body movement. Eye movements began with the infants' slightest stirring and persisted for a little while after the infant became still. Such eye movements had not been studied in adults in any systematic way, so as a logical follow-up to this experiment, Aserinsky and Kleitman set out to perform a similar experiment in adults. The instrumentation was to be much more sophisticated, however. They would record eye movements electrically with small electrode disks glued near the eyes and would also record the EEG, heart rate, respiration, and body movement.

The same eye movements that were seen in the infants were seen in the adults. They were slow, pendular movements, frequently binocularly asymmetrical, which required 3 to 4 seconds for completion. As in the infant, these slow eye movements occurred whenever there was gross body movement. But in addition, for the first time a new type of eye movement was observed. The eyes moved together in rapid jerky motions of relatively short arcs, which were followed by a fixational pause. A single movement was complete in a fraction of a second. These rapid eye movements or REMs occurred in clusters at particular times during sleep. The first period of REMs was seen an hour or so after the onset of sleep and was the shortest such REM period of the night—about ten minutes long. As the night's sleep progressed, three or four more REM periods occurred. The time interval between REM periods grew shorter and the duration of the REM periods longer as the night wore on.

During the REM period there was no gross body movement. Very fine distal limb and finger movements did occur, and these movements were not seen at any other time during the night. The EEG took on a characteristic appearance during the REM period. It was the low-level, irregular signal similar to that recorded during the waking state. REM periods were also characterized by increased heart rate and irregular and rapid respiration. To Aserinsky and Kleitman these physiological changes suggested the sort of emotional disturbance that might be caused by dreaming. In Kleitman's words:

> To test this supposition, sleepers were aroused and interrogated during or shortly after the termination of REMs and they almost invariably reported having dreamed. If awakened in the absence of REMs or when questioned after a night's undisturbed sleep, they seldom recalled dreaming.

It appeared that dreaming occurred during the four or five sequential REM periods of a night's sleep and at no other time.

Perhaps as remarkable as the association of dreaming with episodes of rapid eye movement, fine finger and limb movement, and a low-level random EEG signal was the sequence of neural events in which the REM periods were embedded. Kleitman and a second graduate student, William Dement (currently professor of psychiatry and head of the Sleep Laboratory at Stanford University), recorded the EEG in thirty-three subjects throughout the night without awakening them and found that the confusing array of EEG signals seen by earlier investigators actually occurred in an orderly, cyclic pattern as the night progressed. First they saw the alpha rhythm as the subject closed his eyes in preparation for sleep, then a low-level random signal, similar to the waking state except that now the subject was asleep. They called this state the "descending" stage 1 of sleep.

Some minutes later Dement found the EEG signal changing to a higher amplitude pattern, which he termed stage 2, then to stage 3, and—about a half hour into sleep—to stage 4. Each EEG pattern was distinctive. Large slow waves called delta waves began to appear in stage 3 and filled the record in stage 4. And then the process reversed —back through stages 3 and 2 to "ascending" stage 1, so designated to distinguish it from what turned out to be the unique characteristics of "descending" stage 1 at the beginning of the night. "Ascending" stage 1 was the period during which there were rapid eye movements, so this stage was called the REM stage.

The first REM period was short, an average of 9 minutes for Dement and Kleitman's subjects. Besides the rapid eye movements there was the irregular rapid breathing and the fine finger movements described by Aserinsky. The occurrence of the REM period completed the first sleep cycle. It took about an hour and a half.

The cycle was then repeated three or four more times during the night. The time between REM periods became progressively shorter and the periods themselves progressively longer as sleep continued. The last REM period of the night was 30 or 40 minutes long. In later cycles stage 4 did not occur, and stage 3 was rare. The cycles consisted largely in an alteration between stage 2 and stage REM. All of this is shown in the figure on page 45.

Dement and Kleitman published their findings in 1957. The cyclic EEG patterns they observed have been verified in thousands of sleep records taken since that time. It is clear that all normal individuals experience four or five sleep cycles a night, each ending in a REM period during which dreaming occurs.

At this point an array of questions was asked and, in research continuing to this day, is being answered experimentally to greater or lesser extent. What sort of neuronal activity occurred in the brain, particularly in the forebrain structures such as neocortex and hippocampus, during the various stages of sleep? Was there any meaning to the different EEG patterns seen in the various stages of sleep? What brain mechanisms turned the sleep cycle on and sequenced it in an orderly fashion? How tenacious was the cycle—what would happen if a subject was deprived of one stage of sleep, say REM, by repeated awakenings? Were thought processes of any kind going on in other than REM periods? Although dreaming had not been reported in awakenings from other sleep stages, at least in one stage—descending stage 1 as sleep began—Dement noted dreamlike thoughts. What about dream content itself? Was there any pattern or meaning in the sequential dreams of a given night? Did the dreams of the mentally ill differ from those of normal people? The way was now open to examine all of the dream content of a night, since subjects could be awakened at the end of each REM period to relate content without forgetfulness and possible distortion involved in daytime recall. And lastly, was the cyclic neural process which occurred during sleep unique to man? If not, what was its evolutionary origin—and its function? The answers to some of these questions will be important features of my argument and will bear directly on my hypothesis.

Researchers found that the sleep cycle was present in other mammals as well as in man, and this allowed much to be learned that could not have been learned otherwise. Electrodes could be placed directly within the brains of animals to study the activity of a single neuron or small population of neurons in a specific structure, for example the visual cortex or a lower brain center. Thus the activity of a small part of

44

BRAIN AND PSYCHE

the brain could be monitored during the waking state or in a particular phase of sleep.

Cats were the first experimental animals to be used. Dement identified the sleep cycle in cats a year after his study of humans, and investigations were begun in a number of laboratories. The sleep cycle in cats was shorter than in humans but the stages of sleep were there. The stages preceding REM were not as finely analyzed in cats as in humans —they were all classed as one stage (equivalent to human stages 2, 3, and 4) named slow-wave sleep because the EEG record showed a preponderance of large slow waves. REM sleep looked the same as in humans, characterized by low-level, random EEG, rapid eye movements, and rapid irregular breathing. And in cats, accompanying the rapid eye movements were twitches of the whiskers, ears, paws, and tail. Although the cycles did not last as long, their organization was the same. In a given bout of sleep, a relatively long period of slow-wave sleep was followed by a brief REM period, a few minutes long, and

ILLUSTRATION 8
(Upper)

William Dement and Nathaniel Kleitman found that a distinct series of EEG signals occurs in sequence during a night's sleep. Sleep begins with descending stage 1, a low-level irregular EEG signal similar to that seen in the alert, waking state, but now the subject is asleep. (The initial part of the first record shows alpha rhythm. The subject is lying awake with his eyes shut before falling asleep.) Stage 2, in which the EEG shows larger amplitude components, begins a few minutes later. Stage 3 with a scattering of large delta waves and stage 4 made up largely of such waves follow in sequence. The sequence then reverses, stages 4, 3, 2, and finally ascending stage 1 or the REM stage. This is the sleep stage in which there are rapid eye movements and dreaming.

(Lower)

The sleep cycle repeats itself four or five times during the night. Illustrated is a typical sleep cycle from eleven at night to seven in the morning. The time between REM periods grows progressively shorter and the REM stages progressively longer. Thus, the first REM period may be ten minutes long and the last may take forty minutes. Dement and Kleitman established that the normal human has four or five REM periods each night during which dreaming occurs.

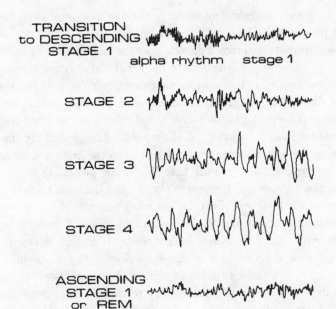

TRANSITION
to DESCENDING
STAGE 1

alpha rhythm   stage 1

STAGE 2

STAGE 3

STAGE 4

ASCENDING
STAGE 1
or REM

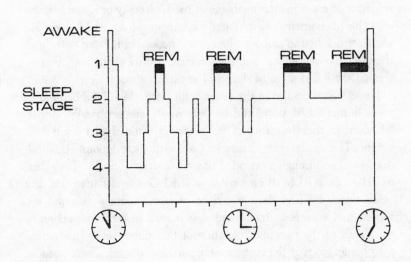

AWAKE

REM   REM   REM   REM

1

SLEEP
STAGE   2

3

4

then there were progressively shorter periods of slow-wave sleep and longer periods of REM.

Now scientists could record directly from the neurons of the neocortex. They found that the neurons of the visual and association cortex (in which information from various senses were combined) were active during REM sleep, at least as active as during the alert, waking state (activity was lower during slow-wave sleep). This was consistent with the low-level EEG seen during REM sleep—the EEG looked the same as during the waking state. During REM sleep the brain was apparently performing some internal task. It was not processing external information—the animal's eyes were closed—and the brain's output to the rest of the body was effectively cut off. There was almost a complete disappearance of muscle tone in the limb and neck muscles and consequently normal body and limb movements as seen during the waking state and occasionally in slow-wave sleep were not possible in REM sleep. The slight twitches of the whiskers, ears, paws, or tail which did occur during REM sleep were presumably faint manifestations of what ordinarily would be full-fledged movements of the animal in response to the firing of neurons in its active brain. Michel Jouvet, professor of experimental medicine at the University of Lyons, discovered this phenomenon of inhibited movement during REM sleep. He was so struck by the paradox of an active neocortex isolated both from the external environment and the muscular control of the body that he termed the REM stage of sleep in the cat paradoxical sleep.

Jouvet found centers in the lower brain stem which inhibited movement during REM sleep, and he destroyed them electrically. Adrian Morrison at the University of Pennsylvania made similar brain-stem lesions. The results were dramatic. Cats with these lesions would fall asleep and go through a period of slow-wave sleep normally. They then would enter a REM sleep period—the EEG would flatten and the other signs of REM sleep would be present. There were rapid eye movements, muscle twitches, and as is normal in cats, contraction of the pupils of the eyes and relaxation of the inner eyelids (nictitating membranes) so that the eyeballs were partially covered. There was also elevated brain temperature and a particular electrical signal (theta rhythm) in the hippocampus, which I will describe later. However, instead of remaining in a sleeping position, the animals with lesions in the inhibitory centers of their brain stems raised their heads to make searching and orienting movements. At times they rose and attacked, appeared to be startled or enraged by invisible objects. Throughout this state, the animals were unresponsive to visual stimuli just as they were in normal REM sleep, and the signs of REM sleep listed above persisted.

It seemed that the cats were dreaming and acting out their dreams. The normal inhibition of muscle tone during REM (atonia) presumably had the function of allowing the brain activity of the dream to proceed without the movement that the same brain activity would produce in the waking state. Researchers found consistent results in man. It was found that, like the neck muscles in the cat, chin muscles in man were atonic during REM sleep and this effect is currently monitored along with the flat EEG and rapid eye movements as an indicator of the REM state. Also, correlations have been reported between the sequences of small limb twitches during REM and the content of dreams reported by subjects awakened immediately after the movements. One might suppose that, were it not for motor inhibition, dreamers would attempt to act out the movements of their dreams.*

Dement looked at every aspect of the new sleep cycle phenomenon. He tried REM sleep deprivation, just as Kleitman had tried total sleep deprivation. To quote his rationale from his report on the subject published in *Science* in 1960:

> Since there appears to be no exception to the nightly occurrence of a substantial amount of dreaming in every sleeping person, it might be asked whether or not this amount of dreaming is in some way a necessary and vital part of our existence. Would it be possible for human beings to continue functioning normally if their dream life were completely or partially suppressed? Should dreaming be considered necessary in a psychological or a physiological sense or both?

In his experiment, Dement allowed eight subjects several nights of undisturbed sleep and then deprived them of most of their REM sleep for five successive nights. He monitored their EEG and eye movements throughout the night as indicators of sleep stages and wakened them as soon as he was sure that they had entered a REM period. He found that if he kept them up for at least three minutes, the sleep cycle would not resume where it left off, but a new one would begin. As the night progressed, the subjects needed more and more awakening to be kept out of REM sleep. This effect mounted on successive nights of deprivation—an average of eleven awakenings were required on the first night, twenty-three on the fifth. The subjects were then allowed five nights of undisturbed sleep. During the control nights at the beginning of the experiment, the duration of REM sleep was about 19 percent of total sleeping time. On the first night of undisturbed sleep after deprivation, the amount of REM sleep was about 50 percent higher, and this apparent compensation for lost REM time (called REM rebound) persisted for several nights thereafter. The amount of sleep in other sleep stages did not change as a result of REM deprivation and control subjects awakened as many times from sleep stages other than REM showed no rebound effect. Dement concluded:

> It is as if the pressure to dream builds up with the occurring dream deficit during successive dream deprivation nights—a pressure which is first evident in the increasing frequency of attempts to dream and then during the recovery period results in the marked increase in total dream time and percentage of dream time.

Dement had found a partial answer to his question concerning the physiological necessity for dreaming. The function of the dream still was not understood—why it was a necessity—but whatever brain mechanism controlled the sleep cycle, it stubbornly insisted on completing its course. With regard to the question of psychological necessity, the answer was negative. Although subjects were variously anxious, or agitated, or tended to overeat during the period of the experiment, no important psychological effects were noted.

Jouvet observed the same physiological effects of REM deprivation in cats. Suppressing REM sleep by an electrical shock, he found it necessary to apply shocks at intervals that grew shorter and shorter until, after a few hours, the animals collapsed into a REM state immediately after the shock. There was subsequent REM rebound. The REM rebound phenomenon has also been reported in other animal species.

These initial discoveries of the sleep cycle and the isolated, active brain generating dreams during REM sleep, led to further questions that were explored during the 1960s. As mentioned earlier, Dement's subjects reported dreamlike states when awakened during descending sleep stage 1, just as they were drifting off to sleep. This finding was confirmed and expanded upon in an extensive study by David Foulkes of the University of Colorado and Gerald Vogel of the University of Chicago Medical School. In descending stage 1 subjects experience visual images and segments of dreamlike material, not as lengthy, storylike, or laden with emotion as dreams but a long way from the realistic thoughts that were in the subject's awareness just before they drifted off to sleep.

Thought processes were also found to occur in non-REM sleep, that is stages 2, 3, and 4 which precede REM sleep in the cycle. In Dement and Kleitman's original study, the material that subjects related upon awakening was classified as a dream only if it contained a detailed dream description. On this basis there was virtually no dreaming except during REM periods. Dreams were reported in about 7 percent of the awakenings during non-REM sleep, but these were ascribed to subjects remembering previous dreams of the night. In later studies, subjects were awakened both from REM and non-REM sleep stages and the reported thought content analyzed. Thought processes were prevalent during non-REM sleep stages, including non-REM stages preceding the first REM period of the night (where such thoughts could not be a memory of a previous dream). Non-REM thought was different from dreaming. It was more like normal thinking, still fanciful but less visually and emotionally vivid than dreams and more concerned with happenings in contemporary waking life. At times, subject matter reported in non-REM sleep appeared in later dreams of the night. This was found by Foulkes and also by Allan Rechtschaffen and associates at the University of Chicago. To quote Rechtschaffen:

On those nights when themes and images persist through both non-REM and REM periods, the dreams do not arise sui generis as psychologically isolated mental productions, but emerge as the most vivid and memorable part of a larger fabric of interwoven mental activity.

The association of thought processes with non-REM sleep has not been established as clearly as that of dreams with REM sleep—depending on the laboratory, some 33–70 percent of awakenings from non-REM sleep have been reported to be accompanied by ongoing thoughts—but it is generally accepted that mental activity of some sort occurs throughout the sleep cycle.

Another area of research, which began in the 1960s and is still under active investigation, concerns the brain mechanisms responsible for controlling and sequencing the sleep cycle. Jouvet and his associates performed the initial experiments and continue to be one of the leading research groups in the area. They have shown that the cycle is controlled from the brain stem, the site of regulation of many basic life-sustaining functions, but the precise control mechanisms are as yet unknown.

It may be well to pause at this point to gain perspective. Sleep, at least its REM stage in which there is dreaming, apparently is used by the brain for a unique type of information processing reflected by the dream. The direction of research has emphasized this aspect of sleep—although it has not as yet arrived at the mechanism or purpose of sleep. What are we to make of our most common experience, our need to sleep when we are tired and our feeling of satisfaction when this need is fulfilled? Kleitman and others sought the answers to these questions in their early work. In the remainder of this chapter we will look at two areas of sleep research that are most likely to yield a deeper understanding of the phenomenon; the development of sleep over the life span and the evolutionary history of sleep.

Newborn infants have both REM and non-REM stages of sleep. The stages are not fully developed but are clearly differentiable. During REM sleep there are the customary bouts of rapid eye movements (not noticed in earlier experiments in which no eye movements were recorded), low-level EEG, and irregular breathing. The inhibition of motor centers is not as complete as in adults—along with eye movements there are grimaces, whimpers, smiles, and twitches of the face interspersed with gross body movements. When there is no such movement, however, muscle tone drops as it does in the adult. During non-REM sleep the EEG is higher and there are slow waves much like stage 2 of adult sleep. There are no bursts of eye movements, breathing is regular and chin muscle tone is higher than in REM sleep. Although the stages of sleep are similar to the adult's, their cyclic organization is different. The sleep cycle is about 50–60 minutes long with activity terminating the cycle (Kleitman noted in early studies that there is a 50–60 minute rest-activity cycle in infants which occurs more or less uniformly over a twenty-four-hour period) and the sequence is not necessarily non-REM followed by REM as in the adult, for REM sleep may follow directly after wakefulness.

Infants sleep about sixteen hours a day and in each sleep cycle spend about half the time in each of the two phases of sleep, so that overall they spend eight hours a day in REM and eight hours a day in non-REM sleep. The sleep cycle gradually matures into the adult pattern. By three to five months of age, when infants are generally awake during the day and asleep at night, REM sleep time is down to six hours while non-REM is still about eight hours, and by two to three years the comparable figures are three hours for REM and eight and one-half hours for non-REM. By five to nine years, REM time is down to about two hours, just about the adult level, while non-REM time is still approximately eight hours. Sleep time then gradually diminishes with age until as adults they reach levels of a little over six hours of non-REM sleep and a little under two hours of REM sleep.

These data were mainly gathered by Howard Roffwarg of Columbia University, Joseph Muzio, and William Dement, who wrote a summary report in 1966. Their findings in humans were later expanded upon by others, and a similar developmental pattern of sleep over the span of life was found in animals. From the results of their studies, Roffwarg and associates conceived of a theory of the function of REM sleep. They were struck by two points: If REM sleep is dreaming sleep, what do newborn infants dream about? And why do they have so much

REM sleep? They provided an observation that might have been thought to cast light on what a newborn infant dreams about, namely:

> In the REM state, newborns display facial mimicry which gives the appearance of sophisticated expressions of emotions and thoughts such as perplexity, disdain, skepticism and mild amusement. We have not noted such nuances of expression in the same newborns when awake.

This would seem to be similar to the emotional content of adult dreams. But they based their hypothesis on the second point—the fact that there is so much REM sleep in infants. I noted earlier that during REM sleep there is a high level of neuronal excitation in the forebrain. Roffwarg and his colleagues suggested that this internally generated excitation was necessary for the normal physiological development of the brain and that the function of REM sleep was to provide this excitation. To quote from their report:

> We have hypothesized that the REM mechanism serves as an endogenous source of stimulation, furnishing great quantities of functional excitation to higher centers. Such stimulation would be particularly crucial during the periods in utero and shortly after birth, before appreciable exogenous stimulation is available to the central nervous system. It might assist in structural maturation and differentiation of key sensory and motor areas within the central nervous system, partially preparing them to handle the enormous rush of stimulation provided by the postnatal milieu, as well as contributing to their further growth after birth.

Thus, Roffwarg felt that the great nervous activity during REM sleep aided the brain to finalize its interconnections, since the brain is not fully developed at birth.

REM sleep in adults was considered more or less a holdover from infancy—a means of maintaining central nervous tone. REM sleep was not considered to play a role in information processing. However, in an outstanding experiment performed recently, Roffwarg provided evidence which leads to precisely the opposite conclusion. In the last section of this book I will relate this experiment as well as my own view of the function of REM sleep both in infants and adults.*

We now turn to the last and perhaps most revealing aspect of sleep, its evolutionary history. Sleep has been studied in a large number of placental and marsupial (those bearing infants in a pouch) mammals, and the sleep cycle has been found in all of them. These mammals include such diverse species as man, chimpanzee, several species of monkey, dog, cat, sheep, mole, mouse, rat, rabbit, squirrel, opossum, and bat. However, the amount of sleep as well as the portion of the sleep cycle that is spent in REM sleep varies from species to species. The guinea pig and rabbit sleep fitfully—REM sleep makes up about 5 percent of the sleep cycle in the guinea pig and 15 percent in the rabbit. Humans and cats sleep about eight hours a day or more, and REM sleep makes up about 25 percent of the sleep cycle. Truett Allison and associates at Yale University, who have done extensive work in the evolution of sleep, relate this variation to the way of life of the individual species. Animals subject to predation tend to sleep less and have a lower percentage of REM sleep, while predators or animals that have secure sleeping places sleep longer and have a higher proportion of REM sleep. In any case, the sleep cycle appears to be universal in placental and marsupial mammals.

There is a third order of mammals, the monotremes. These were the first mammals to evolve from reptilian ancestors some 180 million years ago. The mammalian line that gives rise to marsupial and placentals (including man) diverged from the monotreme line sometime after the monotremes appeared. There are only two living examples of monotremes, the echidna or spiny anteater and the duck-billed platypus now found only in Australia and nearby islands. These animals are undoubtedly mammals, for they maintain constant body temperature, have a four-chambered heart, are hairy, and nurse their young, although like their reptilian ancestors, they hatch their young from eggs. Both are small, shy creatures, under two feet in length and eight pounds in weight. The platypus dives to river bottoms to feed on worms and immature shellfish while the echidna burrows in the forest to feed on ants and termites.

Allison and his colleagues carried out a careful study of sleep in the echidna. The EEG, hippocampal electrical activity, eye movements, neck muscle tone, heart rate, respiration rate, and brain temperature were all measured. The result was clear. The animal was a "good" sleeper, slow-wave sleep appeared frequently, but there was no REM sleep at all. Allison considered whether the lack of REM sleep could be due to the particular specializations of the animal. The echidna, like other burrowing animals, had a poor visual system—even when it was awake, eye movements did not occur often. Perhaps the absence of REM sleep was related to this fact. They studied sleep in the mole, an animal that could not use its eyes at all and was virtually blind, and there was a large percentage of REM sleep. This was also true of the opossum, bat, and mole rat, all of which had poor visual systems. The echidna was a hibernator, but REM sleep was present in other hibernators. The echidna's brain temperature was rather low but the brain

ECHIDNA
The echidna, one of two living monotremes, lives in the forests of Australia and neighboring islands.

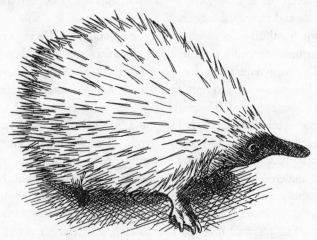

temperatures of the mole and opossum were only slightly higher. Allison concluded that the absence of REM sleep in the echidna was not due to the animal's particular specializations. He concluded that although slow-wave sleep may have arisen with the immediate reptilian ancestors of all the mammals, REM sleep did not; REM sleep first arose about 140 million years ago in a common ancestor of the marsupial and placental mammals after this common ancestor split away from the monotreme evolutionary line.

What can be said about the evolution of slow-wave sleep? A version of slow-wave sleep does exist in turtles, which are distantly related to mammals, and in crocodiles, which are related to birds (birds also have slow-wave sleep). Behaviorally, there are periods of quiescence accompanied by slow-wave activity in the EEG, though the primitive cortex of these animals makes the comparison to the mammalian EEG difficult. The main point relates to temperature. Since reptiles cannot maintain constant body temperature, they are strongly influenced by the temperature of the environment. They become quiescent and their metabolism slows when they are exposed to low temperature. They also become quiescent at high temperatures and can choose this state by moving to sunny locations on their home grounds. Presumably these periods of quiescence and reduced energy consumption form a part of their biological economy.

As just mentioned, turtles and crocodiles are distant reptilian relatives of warm-blooded creatures such as mammals and birds. Possibly in more recent ancestors, or in birds or mammals themselves, slow-wave sleep evolved to provide a period when less energy would be consumed in active movement and thus provide a reserve of energy that could be used to maintain body temperature. In mammals, the cyclic drop in body temperature studied by Kleitman might indicate a nightly slowing of metabolic rate. However, there are no data, and all this is necessarily conjecture.

Research is beginning to shed light on the function of slow-wave sleep in mammals. Experiments suggest that slow-wave sleep may indeed have a restorative effect. Studies of marathon runners have shown a significant increase in slow-wave sleep, especially stages 3 and 4, after a major expenditure of energy in a race. It has also been found that growth hormone is secreted into the bloodstream during the first slow-wave sleep episode of each night's sleep. Growth hormone is known to increase the rate of protein and RNA synthesis suggesting some reparative or restorative role in metabolism. It also promotes body growth during periods of physical development (hence its name). Whether the release of the hormone does in fact initiate a reparative process or whether it is in any way related to our feeling of restored energy after sleep is not known.

And so we would leave our discussion of sleep with a summary—a complex, highly organized cycle of slow-wave and REM sleep occurs throughout the marsupial and placental mammalian kingdom but not in a monotreme, the echidna, where there is no REM sleep—were it not for one additional fact. The echidna has a brain that is entirely out of keeping with its position in phylogeny. It has a huge convoluted prefrontal cortex, a larger prefrontal cortex in relation to the rest of its brain than is possessed by any other mammal including man. This unique aspect of the echidna's brain was described by the anatomist Elliot Smith in 1902:

The most obtrusive feature of this brain is the relatively enormous development of the cerebral hemispheres . . . the extent of the

ILLUSTRATION 9

The prefrontal cortex in each species is shown as a shaded area. For clarity, all brains are drawn to the same size with the relative sizes illustrated below. In placental and marsupial mammals, the amount of prefrontal cortex increases as the animal advances in the mammalian order. In the rat, prefrontal cortex is very small. It grows progressively larger in the cat and monkey, and finally reaches its greatest development in man. The growth of prefrontal cortex is even more pronounced than is shown by the shaded areas, for in higher species the neocortex becomes more and more convoluted, indicating that a greater mass of neural tissue is squeezed together and folded upon itself in a given brain surface area. The brain of the echidna is a remarkable anomaly. Although its behavior and capabilities are no more advanced than those of a rat, it possesses a very large, convoluted prefrontal cortex, greater in size relative to the rest of its brain than any mammal including man.

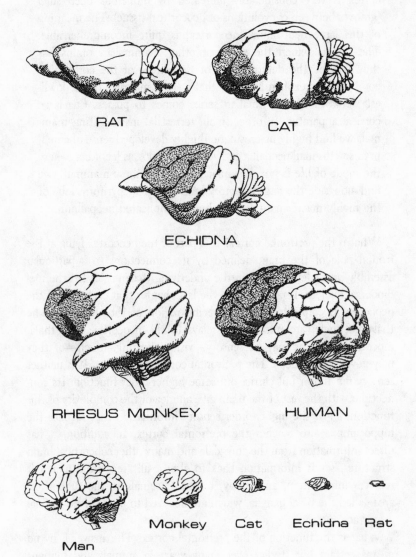

RAT

CAT

ECHIDNA

RHESUS MONKEY

HUMAN

Man

Monkey

Cat

Echidna

Rat

cortex is very considerably increased by numerous deep sulci [grooves between convolutions of neocortical tissue]. The meaning of this large neopallium [neocortex] is quite incomprehensible. The factors which the study of other mammalian brains has shown to be the determinants of the extent of the cortex, fail completely to explain how it is that a small mammal of the lowliest status in the mammalian series comes to possess this large cortical apparatus. In other small, terrestrial insect eating mammals we find highly macrosmatic [highly developed sense of smell] brains with small neopallia and yet in tachyglossus [echidna] where the mode of life is not dissimilar to many of these mammals, we find alongside the large olfactory bulb and great pyriform lobe of the highly macrosmatic brain a huge complicated neopallium.

What is the prefrontal cortex? It is part of the neocortex lying at the frontal pole of the brain defined by its connections to a particular assembly or nucleus of cells in the underlying thalamus called the mediodorsal nucleus. I mentioned in the last chapter that each area of the neocortex is connected with a specific region of the thalamus. The thalamic nuclei are information relays to the neocortex. The thalamocortical systems may be sensory—vision, hearing, touch—or they may govern movement. The prefrontal cortex is different. It is neither sensory nor motor but carries out some higher-order function. Its connections with the rest of the brain give an idea of the complexity of this function; all of the higher-order sensory information that reaches the hippocampus also reaches the prefrontal cortex. In addition, it has direct information from the amygdala and many other subcortical brain structures, sends information back to almost all areas from which it receives information, and, lastly, transmits signals to the subcortical area called the basal ganglia, which are believed to be involved in final motor action.

What is the function of the prefrontal cortex? The answer is by no means certain but studies over many years in animals and humans suggest that the prefrontal cortex may have the task of forming strategies of behavior to achieve a given purpose or goal. To quote from a recent review by Joaquim Fuster of the Brain Research Institute, University of California at Los Angeles, speaking of the synthesis of a behavior:

> The most crucial constituents are the attentive acts that "palpate" the environment in search of significant clues, the intentional and elaborate movements, the continuous updating of relevant information, and the referring of that information to a cognitive scheme of the overall structure and its goal. The prefrontal cortex not only provides the substrate for these operations but imparts to them their active quality. In that active role . . . one may find some justification of the often espoused view of the prefrontal cortex—"the executive of the brain."

This is well illustrated in a report by V. M. Bekhterev, a Russian physiologist, in 1907. He found that lesions of the prefrontal cortex in dogs caused no loss of sensory perception but that such dogs "do not evaluate the results of their actions as they should, cannot correlate new external impressions with past experience and do not direct their movements and actions to their own advantage." In man, damage of the prefrontal cortex also causes a disturbance of the ability to evaluate correctly one's own behavior and actions. There may also be apathy, an indifference to the future, a blunting of affect and emotion or restlessness and impulsive action. In all, prefrontal damage results in a profound change in personality.

What is the echidna doing with this massive prefrontal cortex? Is it in any way related to the fact that the animal does not have REM sleep? In the last section of this book I suggest that there is indeed a relationship and that the echidna's brain constitutes a most significant clue in our endeavor to understand the biological basis of the psyche.

We have now completed the section on Brain. In the first chapter we saw how the brain perceives and remembers, and how, within the limbic system, further functions are performed relating to memory and emotion. In the present chapter the reader was introduced to the processes occurring during sleep and to the prefrontal cortex, which apparently governs the planning of behavior. The psyche is based within these neural processes of the brain. In later chapters we will return to the brain—to the hippocampus, the limbic system, and sleep—to look at neuroscientific discoveries that will give us further clues to psychological function, and then in the last section on Hypothesis, I will gather the clues together and present what I believe is the biological basis of the psyche.

But first, to examine the psychological part of our data, we turn to another world, Vienna, in the middle part of the last century.

Psyche

This book, with the new contribution to psychology which surprised the world when it was published (1900), remains essentially unaltered. It contains, even according to my present-day judgement, the most valuable of all the discoveries it has been my good fortune to make. Insight such as this falls to one's lot but once in a lifetime.

Freud
Vienna
March 15, 1931

Foreword to English translation
of *The Interpretation of Dreams*
by A. A. Brill

Three

THE EARLY DISCOVERIES

Sigmund Freud was a young, gifted, and ambitious medical scientist, a neuroscientist of his day who was drawn to the study of psychological phenomena by the nature of his medical career and by external circumstances. The result was the formulation of a far-reaching theory of unconscious motivation underlying both normal behavior and mental disease—a theory that has engendered controversy since the time of its conception. It has been, and is, viewed by some as the key to understanding man's mental processes and nature, an achievement to be ranked with that of Darwin. By others, as we shall see, it is considered a travesty of science. In this chapter we will trace the manner in which Freud pursued his early career and evolved the ideas that led to the publication in 1900 of *The Interpretation of Dreams*. This will be important later as we attempt to evaluate the significance of his discoveries and theory.

Sigmund Freud was born to a Jewish family in the year 1856 in the town of Freiberg in Moravia, at present a region of East Germany, then a part of the Austro-Hungarian Empire. His father Jacob was forty years old, a trader in cloth. His mother Amalie was twenty, a beautiful young girl whom Jacob had taken as a bride the year before Sigmund's birth. The Freud family—father, mother, Sigmund, and sister Anna, born in 1858—lived very modestly in a single room in the town over a locksmith shop.

In 1859, when Sigmund was three years old, Jacob and his family left Freiberg for Vienna. Jacob was looking for greater opportunities in business. Over the period of the next six years Amalie gave birth to three more daughters and a son. Jacob's fortunes improved so that by the time Sigmund passed the entrance examination for the local *Gymnasium* at the age of nine, the Freud family—father, mother, and six children—occupied a three-bedroom apartment, which also contained a small extra room set off from the rest of the flat. The room was Sigmund's bedroom and study until his middle twenties.

Freud showed his intellectual capacity early. He was at the top of his class at the *Gymnasium* during his first year and remained there until he graduated, summa cum laude, at the age of seventeen. His mother's favorite, clearly gifted academically and personable in appearance and demeanor, the young Freud occupied a privileged position in his family and exerted considerable influence over the lives of his sisters.

When he was graduated from the *Gymnasium*, Freud was faced with the choice of a profession. His interest soon turned to science. Darwin's theory was being widely debated at the time, and Freud's imagination was captured by the challenge of unraveling the secrets of nature. This path led the seventeen-year-old Freud to enroll at the medical school of the University of Vienna in the autumn of 1873. He was not particularly drawn to medicine, but during that period the study of medicine was often used as a means of pursuing a career in the natural sciences.

In the late nineteenth century, the University of Vienna was an international center of learning. Each medical department was headed by a renowned academic physician. Theodor Meynert, head of psychiatry, was Europe's foremost cerebral anatomist; Ernst Brücke, director of the Institute of Physiology, was a widely respected physiologist. Brücke and others were leading the turn from a philosophical to a physiological view of nature; they were convinced that ultimately psychological phenomena could be explained in terms of physiological processes, and physiological processes in turn by physical and chemical laws. There was, in addition, a long tradition of culture in the city of Vienna and at the university. Besides medical subjects and courses in the natural sciences, lectures in philosophy and literature were available to the students. An example was set by the faculty—students following the work of Brücke would find, in addition to scientific papers, writings on the fine arts and German poetry.

The medical course at the university was a minimum of five years, each year divided into two semesters and a summer vacation—similar to curricula at our own universities. The student was allowed considerable freedom. There were certain compulsory courses, but he could register for and attend any other course at the university for which he paid the fee. There were no checks on attendance, no course examinations, or assignments. The sole requirement was that a student pass comprehensive examinations on three medical subject areas during the five-year period. One examination was generally taken at the end of the course of study, the other two sometime before. During the course of study, many students did additional work in the laboratories or hospitals, according to their interests.

Freud received his medical degree on March 31, 1881, at the age of twenty-five, having taken almost eight years to complete his work. During his first two years he followed the required courses plus a few additional ones such as several in logic, Greek philosophy, and psychology and a course in general biology and Darwinism. In his second year, Freud began a concentrated study of the natural sciences, notably zoology, and in his third, settled down to the study of the comparative anatomy of various animal species. At the end of that year, Freud published his first scientific paper, a study of the male sex organs of the eel. Freud then moved to Ernst Brücke's Institute of Physiology where he found a congenial scientific home until his graduation in 1881 and for a year beyond that, a total of six years in all.

At the time that Freud studied medicine, there were three paths to a medical career, not unlike those that may be followed today. One could take five years of courses with an emphasis on clinical studies, gather clinical experience at hospitals during the summers, and then open a general practice. Or one could intern for two or three additional years in a particular clinical area and then practice as a specialist. Alternatively, one could enter academic medicine, concentrating in a scientific or clinical domain, and then slowly and competitively work one's way after two to five years to the rank of *Privatdozent* (unsalaried university lecturer) and beyond that to an appointment as extraordinary (adjunct) or ordinary (full) professor. Freud's natural tendency was to follow the last of these paths, which he did by continuing to work in the Brücke laboratory. He enjoyed the work and was good at it. His specialty was comparative neuroanatomy, the study of the interconnections of neurons within the nervous systems of animals and the changes that had occurred during evolution in these systems. During his tenure at the laboratory, Freud published several scientific papers that were praised by Brücke. He also came to share firmly the belief of the laboratory that all of biology, even psychology, would finally be capable of description in physiological terms. We shall see that, although Freud tried to but could not provide such a description for the psychological phenomena he discovered, he maintained this belief to the end of his life.

Freud's plans for a career changed suddenly in 1882, when he was twenty-six years old. Upon graduation, he had been appointed demonstrator in Brücke's institute at a small salary commensurate with his teaching duties. However, he was barely able to get along financially, having to borrow at times from more well-to-do friends. Although he hoped that in his research he might make a discovery that would establish his reputation (perhaps a new technique for staining brain tissue), unless something of this fortuitous nature occurred, his prospects were dim. The issue was brought to a head by two events. In the June of 1882, Brücke approached Freud and pointed out that, since two young members of the laboratory were senior to him in the line of advancement, it would be prudent for Freud not to count on a scientific career in the laboratory, but to turn to clinical medicine. The second event occurred in April. On returning home from the institute one evening, he met a friend of his sister's, twenty-one-year-old Martha Bernays, and fell in love. Martha was a slim, attractive young woman with a firm character. She was the daughter of a reasonably well-to-do merchant family that had moved to Vienna from Hamburg in 1869. It was love at first sight for Freud, Martha was soon won over, and by June the couple became engaged. According to the custom of the time, marriage could not take place until a couple's finances were adequate, and indeed Freud could not marry until 1886, four years later.

As a consequence of these new circumstances, Freud began in July of 1882 three years' hospital residency from which he would emerge as a specialist in neurology. He found it unsettling to leave science and was unsure of a specialty as he started to work his way through the various departments of the hospital: surgery, internal medicine, and then psychiatry under Meynert. In May 1883, at the age of twenty-seven, he moved to the hospital and never returned to his parents' home again.

In the Department of Psychiatry, aside from his psychiatric residency, he was offered the opportunity to join Meynert's cerebral anatomy laboratory. Although later in his stay at the hospital Freud carried out research in this laboratory studying nerve tracts of the human brain stem, he decided against turning his career in this direction permanently. Psychiatry itself impressed him as an "unfruitful" discipline. Sometime during his psychiatric stint, Freud decided to specialize in neurology, apparently on the basis of his natural affinity for studying the nervous system and the judgment that there was a place for him as a neurologist within the Viennese medical community. He consequently spent fourteen months in the Department of Nervous Diseases, completing his medical training with several months in ophthalmology. Finally in 1885, sponsored by Brücke, Meynert, and Hermann Nothnagel, head of internal medicine, Freud was invited to apply for the position of *Privatdozent* in neuropathology, a highly prized special lectureship which constituted official recognition of his status as a neurologist. Early in the summer of 1885, he gave his trial lecture entitled "The Medullary Tracts of the Brain" and was appointed *Privatdozent* in September of 1885 at the age of twenty-nine.

It is from this point that we may begin to trace the origin of psychoanalysis. In March of 1885 Freud had applied for a traveling fellowship, which was to be awarded competitively and would, if won, allow him a six-month leave and sufficient funds to attend the lectures and demonstrations of the renowned neurologist Jean-Martin Charcot at the Salpêtrière in Paris. In June Freud learned that as the result of the strong support of Ernst Brücke, he had been granted the fellowship, and he prepared enthusiastically for the journey. Starting in August he would visit his betrothed Martha for six weeks in a resort town and then proceed to Paris. Upon his return he planned to open a private practice and perhaps soon be sufficiently well established to marry. His state of mind was expressed in a letter to Martha:

I am coming with money and staying a long time and bringing
something beautiful for you and then go on to Paris and become a
great scholar and then come back to Vienna with a huge, enormous halo and then we will soon get married, and I will cure all
the incurable nervous cases and through you I shall be healthy and
I will go on kissing you till you are strong and gay and happy.

To a young neurologist, the Salpêtrière was the place to be. Physicians from all over the world were attending Charcot's lectures. Freud's
expertise was in the study of brain anatomy, and he expected to continue such studies at the Salpêtrière. But Freud was there to learn all he
could. Charcot's major fame lay in the diagnosis and treatment of
hysteria, a mysterious condition then prevalent predominantly among
women. Freud had encountered cases of hysteria during his residency
and might be expected to meet them frequently in his private practice.
A patient suffering from this malady had been treated by the physician
Josef Breuer several years earlier, and Freud had discussed it in detail
with Breuer at the time. Thus, Freud had no doubt pondered the
etiology of hysteria with its perplexing interplay of physical and mental
symptoms. I will describe Breuer's case, the well known Anna O., before we go on to Freud's experiences in Paris. It is from Breuer's treatment of this patient that psychoanalysis arose.

Josef Breuer was a highly respected medical scientist and physician,
some twelve years older than Freud. The two had met in Ernst
Brücke's laboratory and had become friends while Freud was a medical
student—Breuer was one of those who helped Freud financially. Breuer
came from the same Viennese Jewish community as Freud, worked in
Brücke's laboratory, and had made several important scientific discoveries before turning to the practice of medicine. (He delineated a mechanism involved in the regulation of breathing, the Hering-Breuer reflex,
and the function of the ear's semicircular canals.) Breuer had been
elected a member of the Vienna Academy of Sciences and was considered an especially gifted physician, as was evidenced by the fact that
among his patients were Brücke, other senior members of the medical
faculty, and the Prime Minister of Hungary.

The case of Anna O. (later revealed to be Bertha Pappenheim, twenty-one-year-old daughter of a prominent Jewish family) began in December of 1880. At the time Breuer was summoned to see the patient, she had for a period of seven months been nursing her fatally ill father and then had suddenly developed a series of bizarre symptoms. Breuer described Anna as being under normal circumstances markedly intelligent with penetrating intuition, energetic, and basically kind—altogether an admirable young woman. When Breuer saw her she was severely paralyzed—she could not use her neck muscles to move her head, her right and later her left leg were rigid, as was her left arm. She had no feelings in her legs, she suffered from disturbances of vision and had a severe cough.

In addition, Breuer found that Anna spontaneously displayed two personalities. In her normal state she was melancholy and anxious. In her second state she was abusive and, to whatever extent she could manage it, destructive. If anything occurred in her room while she was in her second state—an object moved or a person entered or left the room—on her return to normal consciousness she would complain that people were trying to mix her up. She did not remember what had transpired.

At this stage of her illness, Anna would fall into a drowsy state of daydreams for several hours every afternoon (she had slept in the afternoon during the time she was nursing her father at night) and would awaken with the words "tormenting, tormenting." Breuer would see the patient in the evening, hypnotize her, and ask her to relate her daydreams. This procedure, which she called her talking cure, began to relieve her symptoms. At a certain point the patient lost control of grammar and syntax and spoke laboriously using four or five languages. Then, as Breuer reported:

> For two weeks she became completely dumb and in spite of making great and continuous efforts to speak she was unable to say a syllable. And now for the first time the physical mechanism of the disorder became clear. As I knew, she had felt very much offended over something and had determined not to speak about it. When I guessed this and obliged her to talk about it, the inhibition, which had made any other kind of utterance impossible as well,

disappeared . . . but thenceforth she spoke only in English [German was her native language]. . . .

On April 1, 1881, after four months of treatment, the paralysis receded sufficiently for Anna to get out of bed.

On April 5, Anna O.'s father died, and she suffered a relapse. There was a violent outburst of excitement followed by two days of stupor. When she awoke, most of her earlier symptoms returned, and she could not recognize faces (Breuer was the sole exception). She had to try to reconstruct faces from individual features, noses, hair, etc., that she did recognize. Breuer resumed her treatment but her condition deteriorated. Anna refused to eat—Breuer had to feed her. Suicidal ideas developed which prompted Breuer to transfer his patient to a private sanatorium (June 1881) where he continued treatment. By the autumn, Anna responded sufficiently so that she was able to return to Vienna to a new house in which her family now lived. Here the split in Anna's personality grew more pronounced, and Breuer reported a remarkable phenomenon. The second personality was reliving in a day-by-day fashion events that had occurred exactly one year earlier. (Breuer was able to check this from a day-by-day diary kept by Anna's mother.) Breuer wrote:

> She was carried back to the previous year with such intensity that in the new house she hallucinated her old room, so that when she wanted to go to the door she knocked up against the stove which stood in the same relation to the window as the door did in the old room. The change-over from one state to another occurred spontaneously but could also be very easily brought about by any sense-impression which vividly recalled the previous year. One had only to hold up an orange before her eyes (oranges were what she chiefly lived on during the first part of her illness) in order to carry her over from the year 1882 to the year 1881.

Treatment continued with slow progress until an incident occurred that led Breuer to change his technique. Anna would not drink water and was living on fruit. Under hypnosis she told Breuer she had seen

her English lady-companion's dog drinking from a glass—"horrid creature"—and had been angry but had held it back. Having said this, still
under hypnosis, she asked for and drank a large quantity of water. After
she awakened, the symptoms vanished never to return. From this time
on, Breuer adopted the method of asking Anna to trace back, while
under hypnosis, in reverse chronological order each time a particular
symptom had appeared (the cathartic method). Thus:

> These findings—that in the case of this patient the hysterical
> phenomena disappeared as soon as the event which had given rise
> to them was reproduced in her hypnosis—made it possible to ar-
> rive at a therapeutic technical procedure which left nothing to be
> desired in its logical consistency and systematic application. Each
> individual symptom in this complicated case was taken separately
> in hand, all the occasions on which it had appeared were described
> in reverse order, starting before the time when the patient became
> bed-ridden and going back to the event which had let to its first
> appearance. When this had been described the symptom was per-
> manently removed.

The last symptom, paralysis of Anna's left arm, was removed when
she remembered that while she was nursing her father on one occasion,
she grew drowsy and hallucinated a black snake. It was approaching her
father, and Anna tried to move her arm to ward it off but could not
(her arm had most likely fallen asleep). She was terrified and said a
prayer in English, the only one that came to her mind. After recovering
the memory, the paralysis disappeared, and she was once again able to
speak in German.

Thus in June of 1882, after one and a half years, Breuer completed
his treatment. He stated in his report of the case in 1895, some thirteen years later, that Anna O. took some time to recover her full
mental balance. According to the historian Frank J. Solloway, Bertha
Pappenheim had to be reinstitutionalized a total of three times, the last
instance being in 1887, five years after treatment with Breuer. However, she did later go on to a productive life, founding the social work
movement in Germany.

From the viewpoint of the development of psychoanalysis, the fact that tracing symptoms back to the time of their first appearance relieved the symptoms, Breuer's cathartic method, suggested to Freud a particular concept of the organization of the mind. For our present purposes, we should note two unusual aspects of hysteria. First is the remarkable control of mind over body, such as the induction of paralysis and disturbances of vision (at times Anna O. suffered such restriction in her visual field that in looking at a bunch of flowers, she could only see one flower at a time). Second is the relative rarity of hysteria today. As contrasted to such mental diseases as schizophrenia, which were clearly identified in Freud's time and whose prevalence and symptoms have been relatively unchanged since, the prevalence of hysteria has undergone marked changes historically. In the 1880s, the condition was Charcot's main preoccupation, the subject of numerous scientific papers, and constituted a substantial portion of Freud's early practice. Yet hysteria and multiple personality are not often seen today. The historian of psychiatry Henri Ellenberger notes that there was a considerable decline in the number of cases after 1900, and indeed there was a change in the nature of hysteria from the 1820s to the 1880s. The dual personality aspects of Anna O.'s case were different from most hysterias of the 1880s (as we shall see later in this chapter) but were similar to cases seen sixty years earlier. We will return to a discussion of these points in the third section of this book, but let us now follow Freud to Paris.

Freud arrived in Paris on October 13, 1885, following his visit with his fiancée and her family. He settled in and did some sightseeing, and then, on October 20, he reported to the Salpêtrière. The Salpêtrière was a large complex of buildings that had been used as a medical poorhouse for several thousand women. In 1870, Jean-Martin Charcot had been given charge of a large section of the complex. He had soon realized the potential of this patient population for the study of neurological disease, and had successfully transformed it into the foremost neurological teaching hospital in Europe. He had come to the study of hysteria through his attempt to distinguish organically based epilepsy from hysterically based epilepsy, a condition of some prevalence at the time. He also studied traumatic hysteria, an outbreak of hysterical symptoms that might occur sometime after an accident. It was apparent in some of these cases, such as hysterical paralysis, that physical damage to the nervous system was not involved since the paralytic symptoms did not correspond to the known neuroanatomy. As Freud stated later, hysteria behaves as if there were no such thing as anatomy of the brain; its distribution is purely ideational.

The vagueness of hysteria was such that physicians were reluctant to treat it. Its cause was unknown, and it was difficult to distinguish from malingering. Charcot provided a legitimacy for hysteria by demonstrating a rationale for its existence, a psychological rather than a neurological one. In one aspect of this demonstration, Charcot studied three men admitted to the Salpêtrière with a paralysis of the arm following an accident. The symptoms did not correspond to those of organic paralysis and were thus presumed to be hysterical. After determining the symptoms of the paralysis, he chose other subjects, easily hypnotized, and suggested under hypnosis that their arms were paralyzed. The symptoms were the same as for traumatic paralytics. He then further demonstrated a model for the effect of trauma by suggesting to subjects under hypnosis that upon awakening, when slapped on the back (the trauma), their arms would become paralyzed. Later, when their backs were slapped in this way, the paralysis did indeed occur, with the same constellation of symptoms. Charcot gave similar demonstrations for cases of hysterical inability to speak. His concept was that following the shock of trauma, the nervous system was in a state analogous to hypnosis and thus subject to "autosuggestion," which induced the hysterical symptom. He further believed that this was not a process that occurred in the normal brain, but required a hereditary predisposition and revealed brain degeneracy. Charcot treated hysteria by commanding or suggesting under hypnosis that the symptoms disappear.

For the first time Freud was exposed directly to the concept that a set of ideas of great potency (those in the hypnotized subjects as well as the hysterics) could exist in the mind without conscious awareness. He wrote later in his autobiography:

I received the profoundest impression of the possibility that there could be powerful mental processes which nevertheless remained hidden from the consciousness of men.

Freud had presented his credentials to Charcot on his first day at the Salpêtrière and made ready to continue his anatomical studies of the brain. However, his imagination was soon taken by what he saw. He wrote to his fiancée in November:

Charcot, who is one of the greatest physicians and whose common sense borders on genius, is simply wrecking all my aims and opinions. I sometimes come out of his lectures as from out of Notre Dame with an entirely new idea about perfection. But he exhausts me; when I come away from him I no longer have any desire to work at my own silly things . . . whether the seed will ever bear any fruit, I don't know; but what I do know is that no other human being has ever affected me in the same way.

After four months in Paris, during which he observed, and also translated a series of Charcot's lectures into German, Freud returned to Vienna in February of 1886 to open a practice and to marry.

Before proceeding with the next series of events which led to the development of psychoanalysis, it will be valuable for our future understanding to consider briefly the histories of hysteria and hypnotism. Henri Ellenberger provides the following summary with regard to hysteria:

For twenty-five centuries, hysteria [named by the Greeks for *hystera*, the uterus] had been considered a strange disease with incoherent and incomprehensible symptoms. Most physicians believed it to be a disease proper to women and originating in the uterus. Starting in the sixteenth century, some physicians claimed that its seat was in the brain and that it could occasionally be found in men also. A truly objective and systematic study of hysteria [began] with the French physician Briquet, whose celebrated *Traité de l'Hystérie* was published in 1859. . . . Within ten years and with the help of his staff, he made an investigation of 430 hysterical patients. He defined hysteria as "a neurosis of the brain, the manifestation of it consisting chiefly in a perturbation of those vital acts which are concerned with the expressions of emotions

and passions." He found one case of male hysteria for twenty cases
of female hysteria. Briquet absolutely denied the then commonly
held view of erotic cravings or frustrations as being at the root of
this disease (he found hysteria almost non-existent among nuns,
but very frequent among Paris prostitutes). He attached much
importance to hereditary factors (he found that 25 per cent of the
daughters of hysterical women became hysterical themselves). He
further found that hysteria was more common in the lower social
classes than in the higher strata of society, more frequent in the
country than in the city, and he concluded that hysteria was
caused by the effect of violent emotion, protracted sorrows, family
conflicts, and frustrated love, upon predisposed and hypersensitive
persons. Charcot was later to take over the main lines of this
concept of hysteria.

The incoherence and incomprehensibility of the symptoms of hysteria were due to the fact that it was ideas, with their immense diversity,
rather than the anatomical structure of the nervous system, that determined the symptoms. Thus symptoms could include anything the hysterical patient had witnessed or imagined. A dramatic example was
hysterical epilepsy, Charcot's original subject of interest at the Salpêtrière, where the symptoms might have been derived from events the
patients had seen or ideas the patient had gathered from another
source.
Not infrequently (but certainly not always) associated with hysteria
was the condition of multiple personality. This was one feature of the
case of Anna O. A small number of more dramatic cases of multiple
personality, some with and some without marked hysterical symptoms,
have been reported from the beginning of the nineteenth century to
the present. Such patients exhibit, successively, two or more distinct
personalities. Each may go by a different name, speak in different accents or different languages, possess different skills, and each personality may conceive of itself as being of a different chronological age. Each
personality may or may not know of the existence of the others. The
onset of the multiple personalities may be brought on by a trauma.
Among the historical examples, Ellenberger cites the case of a twelve-

year-old Swiss girl, Estelle, who suffered severe paralysis following a fall. She was brought to the French physician Despine in 1836. Despine suspected elements of dual personality and began treating the girl with hypnosis.

In the normal state she was still paralyzed. The slightest movement caused her intolerable pain. She had to be covered with cushions, blankets, eiderdown blankets; she loved her mother and demanded her constant presence, she addressed Despine respectfully with *vous*. In her magnetic [hypnotized] state, she became able to move, started to walk, felt a craving for snow and could not tolerate her mother's presence; she addressed Despine in the familiar way with *tu*.

Within a month of treatment, Estelle began spontaneously taking on alternate personalities. In one she was unable to take a single step. In the other she would walk, run, and loved to play with snow. The young girl became dependent on Despine. Over a six-month period he gradually reduced this dependence and effected a fusion of the personalities in which the symptoms disappeared.

Several patients with multiple personalities were reported by Pierre Janet, a philosopher, psychologist, and physician who was Freud's contemporary. Janet worked first at Le Havre and then at the Salpêtrière and had independently come upon the cathartic method in treating hysteria.

In the same era, Morton Prince, American psychiatrist, reported the case of Christine Beauchamp. Miss Beauchamp first saw Prince in 1898. She was twenty-three years old, well educated, of high moral character, and timid. She complained of headaches, fatigue, and a lack of will. Miss Beauchamp's mother had died when the girl was thirteen, and she had suffered several psychic shocks shortly thereafter. Prince began to treat her with hypnosis and soon found two new subpersonalities emerging. The first was a stricter version of the normal patient while the second, who called herself Sally, was the opposite—gay, reckless, and rebellious. Sally could not speak French, as did Miss Beauchamp, and frequently stuttered. The normal Miss Beauchamp did not know of the existence of her subpersonalities. Sally knew Miss Beauchamp, whom she considered stupid, as well as the other subpersonality (called B II by Prince). B II knew Miss Beauchamp but not Sally.

After several months of treatment, Sally began to emerge without hypnosis, taking over for periods of time and leaving Miss Beauchamp confused and embarrassed by acts Sally had carried out, unbeknownst to her. A fourth, regressed personality appeared sometime later. Over a six-year period, Prince managed to fuse these personalities successfully into one.

A number of other cases of multiple personality have been reported since the turn of the century. Two current examples are the woman described in the book and motion picture *The Three Faces of Eve* and Billy Milligan, a man incarcerated in Ohio for the crime of rape, who exhibits twenty-four personalities, each distinct in name, accent, and behavioral traits.

Woven throughout the history of hysteria and multiple personality is the phenomenon of hypnotism. Hypnotism was first discovered in 1774 by the physician Anton Mesmer in Vienna. Hearing that English physicians were treating certain diseases with magnets, he had a patient swallow a fluid containing iron and then applied magnets to parts of her body. It appeared that her symptoms were relieved. The patient thought that she felt a mysterious fluid running through her body during the treatment. Mesmer concluded that the mysterious fluid responsible for his patient's recovery was present throughout the universe, including man. He then came to see that the swallowing of iron and the use of magnets was not necessary to effect a cure; he was able to relieve patients of their symptoms by touching them, looking into their eyes, and waving his hand over the afflicted part of their body. Mesmer believed he was achieving his results by his own "animal magnetism," which manipulated the mysterious fluid in his patients' bodies.

Mesmer moved to Paris in 1778, where for a period of years he caused a national sensation by treating hundreds of patients, creating a cult, and striving to sell his discovery to the French government. The result was a commission of inquiry appointed by the king in 1784, which prohibited the practice of animal magnetism.

In about 1780, one of Mesmer's followers, the Marquis de Puységur, realized that the real effect of animal magnetism, when it did occur, lay in the psychological effect that the magnetizer, an authority figure, had on the patient and on the magnetizer's power of persuasion (the essence of hypnotism). The phenomenon was given the name "hypnotism" in 1840 by James Braid in England. Although looked on askance by the medical profession from the time of its discovery until about 1880, and three times rejected as a legitimate technique by the French Academy of Sciences, its effects were recognized in certain instances, such as in the treatment of young Estelle by Despine. It was a personal triumph for Charcot that, as a result of his work, the Academy recognized hypnotism in 1882.

I have brought hysteria, multiple personality, and hypnotism to the attention of the reader for several reasons. First, these phenomena are the background from which psychoanalysis arose. Second, I wish to note for our later consideration that any explanation of the functioning of man's mind must take these phenomena into account. Third, they serve to illustrate the difficulties inherent in psychological observations and their interpretation.

Indeed, as the Salpêtrière was in its ascendency, a rival school of hypnotism was being formed at Nancy under the leadership of the physician Hippolyte Bernheim. In contrast to Charcot, who believed that hypnotism was a pathological condition, responsible for the occurrence of hysteria via autosuggestion, which could be used in its treatment, Bernheim stated that hypnotism was a general phenomenon, a state of enforced suggestibility (the current view). Bernheim used hypnosis to treat a variety of disorders and in time came to use it less and less, substituting suggestion in the waking state. Bernheim held that the effects seen at the Salpêtrière were artifacts.

As a matter of fact, certain of the dramatic hysterical epileptic attacks did turn out to be artifactual. Charcot died in 1893, and it was found soon afterward that, unbeknownst to him, members of his staff were in the habit of coaching his star patients so as to please the master. Perhaps more important, the patients themselves, with the dependency that hypnotism and the physician-patient relationship brings, and having observed genuine epilepsy in other patients, may have produced these symptoms without conscious awareness. In addition, without the electroencephalogram as an aid to diagnosis, Charcot may have diagnosed as hysterical epilepsy cases that were real epilepsy caused by lesions of the brain. After Charcot's death, the Salpêtrière turned away from his theories and from hypnotism. The artifacts may have been excused, but as Freud was soon to find in his practice, the use of hypnosis to command or suggest that hysterical symptoms disappear (Charcot's method) was not generally effective.

Freud returned to Vienna in 1886 and, in the spring of that year at the age of thirty, opened his medical practice as a specialist in neuropathology. During the next ten years he would marry, raise a family, establish a substantial medical practice, and develop a new theory of the organization of the human mind.

Freud soon began to achieve a reputation as a specialist in the treatment of hysteria. An important source of patients was Josef Breuer. Breuer's treatment of Anna O. had made it clear to him that he could not, within his time schedule, treat patients of this type. Ernest Jones, Freud's biographer, suggests that Breuer was also uncomfortable with sexual fantasies that Anna O. had developed about him and thus was reluctant to repeat such treatments. In any case, Breuer gladly referred hysteric patients to his younger friend Freud.

Freud began treating hysterics with the medically accepted methods of the time, electrotherapy (the application of electrodes and the passing of a mild current through the body, as described by Wilhelm Heinrich Erb, a German neurologist), baths, massage, and rest. He confined himself to these methods for over a year although his results were largely unsatisfactory. One wonders why Freud did not immediately apply Breuer's cathartic method. Jones suggests that Freud may have been influenced by Charcot's derogatory attitude toward the method when Freud mentioned it to him in Paris. And there was every reason for a new practitioner to use conventional means of treatment. Freud later described in his autobiography his experience with Erb's method during this period:

Unluckily I was soon driven to see that following these instructions was of no help whatever and that what I had taken for an epitome of exact observations was merely the construction of phantasy. The realization that the work of the greatest name in German neuropathology had no more relation to reality than some "Egyptian" dreambook, such as is sold in cheap bookshops, was painful, but it helped to rid me of another shred of the innocent faith in authority from which I was not yet free.

Freud turned to hypnotism as practiced by Charcot in 1887. Outside France, the method was taken seriously by some, but denigrated by others. Meynert wrote that hypnotism "degrades a human being to a creature without will or reason and only hastens his nervous and mental degeneration." Freud did achieve some success with hypnotism, but the results were inconsistent. At times he could not hypnotize his patients at all, and at other times the hypnotic trance was not deep enough for his needs. When a hysterical patient was relieved of her symptoms, the relief was generally temporary.

In search of an improvement of his technique, Freud persuaded a patient whom he had found resistant to hypnotism to accompany him to Nancy, where Bernheim was known to have treated thousands of patients by suggestion under hypnosis. Bernheim was also unable to hypnotize Freud's patient and admitted to him that virtually all of his successes were achieved with poorer and more dependent hospital patients and not with those he saw in private practice. Bernheim further told Freud of an important finding. The hypnotic state was accompanied by amnesia, but Bernheim was able to bring back the memory of events that happened during hypnosis by waking the patient and exhorting the patient to remember while applying pressure to the patient's forehead. This suggested to Freud the possibility that under certain circumstances, his hysteric patients might be made to recall forgotten trauma that might be responsible for their hysterical symptoms.

Freud turned to Breuer's cathartic method around the time of his trip to Nancy. Ellenberger suggests that his interest in the method may have been revived by Pierre Janet's published report of the cathartic cure of a severe case of hysteria in the patient Marie. In any event, in 1899 Freud used the cathartic method to treat Frau Emmy von N.

Frau Emmy von N. was Fanny Moser, widow of a wealthy Swiss indus-
trialist who was referred to Breuer for the treatment of a series of
hysterical symptoms that had begun some years earlier with the death
of her husband. Her symptoms included compulsive twitching and
emitting of sounds, loss of appetite, hallucinations, and animal phobias.
Breuer treated Mrs. Moser first and then turned her over to Freud.
Under hypnosis, the patient recalled a number of traumatic incidents
in her adult life and associated these with earlier incidents in childhood
and with particular symptoms (her animal phobias apparently arose
from her brothers and sisters throwing dead animals at her at the age of
five). Freud treated the patient for seven weeks. Certain symptoms
were relieved, but she was not cured. Freud was to state of this case:

> The therapeutic success on the whole was considerable; but it was
> not a lasting one. The patient's tendency to fall ill in a similar way
> under the impact of fresh traumas was not got rid of. Anyone who
> wanted to undertake the definitive cure of a case of hysteria such
> as this would have to enter more thoroughly into the complex of
> phenomena than I attempted to do.

Mrs. Moser had an unusual ability to recall earlier events and spontaneously reminisced at length, revealing to Freud a glimpse of what later
was to be termed free association.

Fräulein Elisabeth von R., a twenty-one-year-old girl treated in 1892,
could not be hypnotized. Freud turned to Bernheim's pressure or con-
centration technique to have her recall forgotten memories. To quote
Ernest Jones:

> This was the method. The patient, lying down with closed eyes,
> was asked to concentrate her attention on a particular symptom
> and to try to recall any memories that might throw light on its
> origin. When no progress was being made Freud would press her
> forehead with his hand and assure her that then some thoughts or
> memories would indubitably come to her. Sometimes in spite of
> that nothing would seem to happen even when the pressure of the
> hand was repeated. Then perhaps on the fourth attempt, the pa-

tient would bring out what had occurred to her mind, but with the comment: "I could have told you that the first time, but I didn't think it was what you wanted." Such experiences confirmed his confidence in the device, which indeed seemed to him infallible.

The technique of free association developed quite naturally and rapidly to its final form. The patient was asked to lie on a couch, Freud sitting behind her (most early patients were women), and relate all thoughts that came to her mind, regardless of how trivial, embarrassing, or offensive they might be. I will return to the technique and its use in subsequent chapters.

In 1892 and 1893 Breuer and Freud published their first clinical experiences and theoretical comments on hysteria. In 1895, *Studies on Hysteria* appeared in which they related five case histories of patients treated by the cathartic method, Anna O., Frau Emmy von N., Fräulein Elisabeth von R., and two others. All were instances of hysterical symptoms following psychological trauma. The basic finding was that hysterics suffer from memories unavailable to conscious recall. In 1896, on the basis of the treatment of eighteen hysterics, Freud proposed a complex structure of mental organization to account for the unavailability of the memories. The occasion was a lecture before the Viennese Society of Psychiatry and Neurology. The content of the lecture was then published as *The Aetiology of Hysteria*. Freud stated that the trauma that precipitated the most recent outbreak in hysterics was not the basic source of the difficulty. Tracing the incident back through intertwining associated memories, one arrived at particular memories during puberty that were causal. These did not yet fully explain the hysterical condition, however. The ultimate source lay in early childhood, before the age of eight, at which time sexual experiences, generally seduction by an adult, had provided the groundwork for the outbreak later in life. An essential mechanism in the neurosis was repression. The psychic pain of the sexual incident had caused the ego to repress the memory as a means of defense. In Freud's own words:

If we subject a large number of symptoms in many people to this analysis [Breuer's method as now conducted by Freud] we shall come to know of a correspondingly large number of traumatically operative scenes. We have learnt to recognize in these experiences the efficient causes of hysteria; hence we may hope to discover from the study of these traumatic scenes by what influences and in what ways hysterical symptoms are produced. . . .

Tracing an hysterical symptom back to a traumatic scene assists our understanding only if the scene in question fulfils two conditions—if it possesses the required *determining quality* [logical relation to the symptom] and if we can credit it with the necessary *traumatic power*. . . .

Now let us consider to what extent the traumatic scenes of hysteria which are revealed in analysis fulfill the two above requirements in a large number of symptoms and cases. Here we encounter our first great disappointment. It does sometimes happen that the traumatic scene in which the symptom originated really possesses both properties which we require in order to understand the symptom: determining quality and traumatic force. But far oftener—incomparably so—we find realized one of three other possibilities which are very difficult to understand: either the scene indicated by the analysis in which the symptom first made its appearance seems to us not qualified to determine the symptom, for its content bears no relation to the form of the symptom; or the ostensibly traumatic experience whose content is so related proves to be a normally harmless impression, one which ordinarily would have no effect; or finally the "traumatic scene" disconcerts us in both directions, appearing both harmless and altogether unrelated to the peculiar forms of the hysterical symptom. . . .

Moreover, the first disappointment in the practice of Breuer's method is followed immediately by another which must be specially grievous to the physician. Such derivations as these which do not contribute to our understanding of the case in respect of determining quality on traumatic force are also of no therapeutic advantage; the patient keeps his symptoms unaltered. . . .

Freud goes on to state that if one probes beyond these traumatic experiences, one finds a chain of associations leading to earlier trauma of a sexual nature. Thus:

> At first the memory-chains are distinct from one another as they lead backwards, but they branch out; from a single scene two or more memories may be reached at the same time, and from there again there issue side chains the single linking of which may in their turn be joined by association to the links of the main chain . . . the most important result arrived at by a consistent pursuit of analysis is this: whatever the case and whatever symptom we take as our starting point, *in the end we infallibly come to the realm of sexual experience.* So here for the first time we would seem to have discovered an aetiological condition of hysterical symptoms.

These sexual experiences generally occurred around the age of puberty. They were still not the underlying cause of the hysterical symptoms. The key lay in earliest childhood memories. Thus:

> When we are persevering enough to carry our analyses back into early childhood, to the very furthest point which human memory can reach, we thereby in every instance cause the patient to reproduce the experiences which, on account both of their special features and of their relation to the subsequent morbid symptoms must be regarded as the aetiology for which we are looking. These *infantile* experiences are once more *sexual* in content, but are far more uniform in kind than was the case in the scenes of puberty which we had lately discovered; it is now no longer a question of sexual thought being awakened by a chance sensory impression, but of sexual experiences undergone by the patient personally, of sexual intercourse (in the wide sense). You will admit that the importance of such scenes needs no further argument; to this you may now add that in the details of this scene you can invariably discover the determining factors which were perhaps lacking in

those other scenes that had taken place later and were reproduced earlier. . . .

I put forward the proposition, therefore, that at the bottom of every case of hysteria will be found one or more experiences of premature sexual experience which may be reproduced by analytic work though whole decades have intervened. I believe this to be a momentous revelation, the discovery of a *source of the Nile* of neuropathology. . . .

Freud went on to assure his listeners of the care he had taken not to force these recollections of childhood trauma on his patients. The traumata were in the nature of sexual abuses by adults such as servants, teachers, or parents or sexual activities among siblings. Freud set the age of eight as a demarcation point. "Anyone who has not had sexual experiences before this cannot be disposed to hysteria after this; anyone who has had them is ready to develop hysterical symptoms."

He then discussed the important concepts of repression and defense:

But I may also remind you that I myself a few years ago indicated a factor hitherto but little remarked, to which I ascribe the leading part in the production of hysteria *after* puberty [publications of 1893 and 1895]. At that time I put forward the view that the outbreak of hysteria may almost invariably be traced to a *psychic conflict*, arising through an unbearable idea having called up the *defenses* of the ego and demanding repression. In what circumstances this attempt at defense has the pathological effect of actually thrusting into the unconscious a painful memory to the ego and creating an hysterical symptom in its place I could not at that time say. I can complete my statement today. The defense achieves its purpose of thrusting the unbearable idea out of consciousness, if in the (hitherto normal) person concerned, infantile sexual scenes exist in the form of unconscious memories and if the idea to be repressed can be brought into logical or associative connection with any such infantile experience.

Freud finally closed his lecture with the following statement in which he introduces the concept of the unconscious:

I have now come to the end of my subject for today's discussion. I am prepared for contradiction and unbelief, and will therefore say one more thing in support of my position. Whatever you may think of my conclusions, I have the right to ask you not to look upon them as the fruit of idle speculation. They are based on laborious individual examination of patients, which in most cases has taken a hundred or more hours of work. Even more important to me than your estimation of my results is the direction of your attention to the method I have used, which is novel, difficult to handle and yet irreplaceable for scientific and therapeutic purposes. I am sure you will realize that one cannot gainsay the conclusions reached by the use of the modification of Breuer's original method if one neglects that method and uses only the ordinary one of questioning the patient. To do so would be like trying to refute the discoveries of histological technique by the aid of macroscopic investigations. Since the new method of research gives access to a new element in psychic processes, namely, to that which remains unconscious or, to use Breuer's expression, is *incapable of entering consciousness*, it beckons to us with the hope of a new and better understanding of all functional mental disturbances. I cannot believe that psychiatry will long hold back from this new path to knowledge.

I have presented extended excerpts from Freud's 1896 lecture to give the reader a closer idea of his reasoning on the question of hysteria and unconscious mental processes. In passing you may note his singularly elegant and persuasive writing style. I will discuss Freud's views of unconscious processes in the next chapter after seeing their further elaboration in *The Interpretation of Dreams,* but for now let me turn to a consideration of how Freud approached scientific problems—his scientific style.

Freud consistently reached for the broad, encompassing theory. An example was his theory of hysteria which he considered the "source of the Nile" of neuropathology. This propensity of Freud's stemmed from his belief, as a scientist in the Brücke tradition, that there were basic causal mechanisms underlying mental function. Freud looked for these mechanisms as he analyzed his patients. Freud was also ambitious—he wrote to Martha that he would come back to Vienna from Paris, become a great scholar, and cure all the incurable nervous cases. Further, he was concerned with priority of discovery. He wrote to a friend Fliess before his presentation of his sexual theory of hysteria that he had picked up a recent book of Janet's "with a beating heart, and laid it down again with my pulse returned to normal. He has no inkling of the clue. . . ." (Incident related by Freud biographer Ronald W. Clark.) This constellation of characteristics was and is certainly not unusual in a scientist—it is the stuff from which many scientific discoveries are made. The danger, however, is that these characteristics may lead to the formulation of overgeneralized or otherwise incorrect hypotheses which may, for one reason or another, not be corrected by further observations. The danger is especially great in psychology, where observations may be interpreted in a number of alternative ways.

In the matter of hysteria, Freud's conviction that its sole source was childhood sexual trauma led to his minimizing what was apparently an exception to his theory, the case of Anna O., and to a personal estrangement from Josef Breuer. Freud's theory of hysteria also contained a serious error, later corrected, which I will relate below. I will suggest in the third section of this book that another theory formulated by Freud, the wish fulfillment theory of dreams, failed to capture the essence of the function of dreams and that his attempt to interpret all dreams within this framework led to further theories that were unproductive.

Freud's interpretation of the case of Anna O. underwent a metamorphosis between 1892 and 1896. In June of 1892 he wrote a letter to Breuer to give his ideas of what a forthcoming joint publication on hysteria should contain.

We have arrived at our opinions on hysterical attacks by treating hysterical subjects by means of hypnotic suggestion and by questioning them under hypnosis and thus investigating their psychical processes during the attack. Before proceeding to state our views, we must point out that we consider it essential for the explanation of hysterical phenomena to assume the presence of a dissociation —a splitting of the content of consciousness.

This viewpoint did then appear in the joint paper "On the Psychical Mechanism of Hysterical Phenomena" in 1892:

Indeed, the more we occupied ourselves with these phenomena the more certain did our conviction become that that splitting of consciousness, which is so striking in the well-known classical cases of *double conscience* [multiple personalities], exists in a rudimentary fashion in every hysteria and that the tendency to this dissociation—and therewith to the production of abnormal states of consciousness, which may be included under the term "hypnoid" is a fundamental manifestation of this neurosis.

Of course, the case of Anna O. was of this nature. By 1895, Freud apparently considered that Anna O. was an unusual case, an exception to the general rule. In *Studies on Hysteria* published in that year he stated that he had never himself treated such a patient (the four cases reported by Freud in this work did not exhibit hypnoid states or double consciousness), but he agreed that there was such a category. Anna O. differed from Freud's patients in another respect; in her cathartic cure she showed little or no defense. Freud wrote in *Studies on Hysteria:*

I regard this distinction as so important that, on the strength of it, I willingly adhere to this hypothesis of there being a hypnoid hysteria.

But in *The Aetiology of Hysteria* in 1896 he was attempting to force the case of Anna O. into his theory of childhood sexual trauma:

You might think that those rare instances in which analysis can trace the symptom immediately to a traumatic scene of satisfactory determining quality and traumatic force and, by so tracing it, at the same time remove it (as described in Breuer's history of the case of Anna O.) would surely constitute powerful objections to the general validity of the conclusion just propounded. Certainly it looks as if that were so; but I can assure you I have the best of reasons for assuming that even in these cases there exists a chain of operative memories which stretches far back behind the traumatic scene, even though the reproduction of the latter alone may result in the removal of the symptom.

Freud may have been correct—his reasons were not put forth—but it is likely that the condition of double consciousness did and does represent a distinct mental state which may have its own etiology. Indeed, it appears that three constellations may occur: hysteria with multiple personality (Anna O.), hysteria without multiple personality (as emphasized by Freud), and multiple personality without overt hysterical symptoms (Miss Beauchamp, Eve in *The Three Faces of Eve*, and Billy Milligan).

Breuer supported Freud's view of the importance of sexuality in the etiology of hysteria but not to the extent of its causal nature in every case. Thus, he wrote in *Studies on Hysteria:*

It is self-evident and also sufficiently proved by our observations that the non-sexual affects of fright, anxiety and anger lead to the development of hysterical phenomena. But it is perhaps worth while insisting again and again that the sexual factor is by far the most important and the most productive of pathological results.

Breuer's remarks at a discussion of his and Freud's theories of hysteria in 1895 included the remark that the theories they were presenting were provisional and that every theory is a temporary structure.

By 1897, Freud and Breuer were estranged over this issue. The reason for this personal estrangement seemed to be based, as other estrangements were later, on Freud's devotion to his scientific ideas. In a letter to a colleague, Auguste Forel in 1907 (brought to light by scientist-historian Paul F. Cranefield), Breuer wrote:

The case of Anna O., which was the germ-cell of the whole of psycho-analysis, proves that a fairly severe case of hysteria can develop, flourish and be resolved without having a sexual basis. I confess that the plunging into sexuality in theory and practice is not to my taste. But what have my taste and my feeling about what is seemly and what is unseemly to do with the question of what is true?

I have already said that personally I have now parted from Freud entirely, and naturally this was not a wholly painless process. But I still regard Freud's work as magnificent: built up on the most laborious study in his private practice and of the greatest importance—even though no small part of its structure will doubtless crumble away again.

Freud, on his part, believed that Breuer had abandoned his scientific ship.

By 1897, Freud realized that he had made a serious error. He had come to see that the childhood seductions reported by his patients were not true—they were fantasies.

I was at last obliged to recognize that these scenes of seduction had never taken place, and that they were only phantasies which my patients had made up or which I myself had perhaps forced upon them.

The realization developed from several sources. As more and more patients reported childhood sexual abuse, it seemed less and less credible that such abuse was so widespread. Perhaps more important, Freud detected signs of neurosis in one of his sisters. According to his theory that childhood sexual trauma always underlay neurosis (by this time he had expanded his theory to include all neuroses), this would make his father the child molester, an allegation he did not believe. Freud was also analyzing his own dreams at this point and was finding in them childhood sexual fantasies. He wrote later:

Analysis had led back to these infantile sexual traumas by the right path, and yet they were not true. . . . At that time I would have gladly given up the whole work. . . . Perhaps I persevered only because I no longer had any choice and would not then begin at anything else.

From this low point, however, Freud returned three years later to publish *The Interpretation of Dreams,* the source of his greatest discoveries.

Four

THE INTERPRETATION OF DREAMS

By 1895, Freud was completely immersed in psychoanalysis—he was analyzing eight to ten patients a day, six days a week. His patients were using free association to help recover their repressed memories, and some of them brought up their dreams in the course of their associations. Freud soon sensed the presence in these dreams of the unconscious material that he believed was central to his patients' neuroses—the dreams had an uncanny way of getting to the psychological point. In describing this realization some thirty years later, Freud wrote:

> I myself found it [the analysis of dreams] a sheet-anchor during those difficult times when the unrecognized facts of the neuroses used to confuse my inexperienced judgement. Whenever I began to have doubts of the correctness of my wavering conclusions, the successful transformation of a senseless and muddled dream into a logical and intelligible mental process in the dreamer would renew my confidence of being on the right track.

Thus far Freud had only dealt with the dreams and unconscious mental processes of neurotic patients. He wondered how these might differ from the dreams and unconscious processes of normal persons, and so began analyzing his own dreams as well as collecting and studying the dreams of a few friends and colleagues. Freud depended on his patients' free associations to arrive at the meaning of their dreams. Free association is a difficult procedure—relatively few individuals undergoing psychoanalysis today can successfully accomplish it. Self-analysis, the analysis of one's own dreams without the benefit of verbal free association or the help of a psychoanalyst in decoding one's dreams is more difficult still. The danger is that important aspects of a dream's meaning may be lost. Freud himself observed:

> In self-analysis the danger of incompleteness is particularly great. One is too soon satisfied with a part explanation, behind which resistances may easily be keeping back something that is more important perhaps.

(Despite this cautionary comment, we shall later see a striking example of this very problem arising in Freud's self-analysis.)

Freud's self-analysis proceeded over a period of several years. He was deeply affected by the death of his father in 1896—unconscious material concerning his father and his childhood came up in his dreams and was analyzed. By 1899, based on the analysis of his own dreams and those of his patients, Freud had formulated a comprehensive theory of dreams and unconscious mental processes, which appeared in *The Interpretation of Dreams* in 1900. I will summarize the basic concepts of this theory briefly before examining Freud's presentation of it in more detail.

In his theory of the etiology of hysteria, Freud had postulated an unconscious realm of the mind in which traumatic memories of childhood seduction were held, repressed so that they were not available to conscious recall. In *The Interpretation of Dreams*, Freud concluded that dreams reflected memories, fantasies, and desires in the unconscious mind, similarly repressed. The repression occurred because the memories, fantasies, and desires were unacceptable to the conscious mind— they were too shameful or painful to contemplate. Freud believed that during sleep the repression was relaxed, and these repressed ideas surfaced and were expressed in dreams. The repression was not wholly relaxed, however—a censor stood between the unconscious and conscious parts of the mind, disguising the meaning of the dream. But the disguise could be penetrated through the use of free association to arrive at the dream's meaning. That meaning was in every case the fulfillment of an unconscious wish—a wish achieved regardless of its generally perverse consequences. As an example, a childhood wish to have a sibling die and thus gain the undivided love of the mother might be repressed in the unconscious and, either in childhood or in adult life, might form the basis of a dream. Other wishes expressed in dreams might be related to adult concerns but were then always found to be associated with repressed early childhood wishes of an unacceptable nature. Most, though not all, dreams had a sexual content.

Freud believed that the set of repressed unconscious ideas revealed by dreams was instrumental in determining important aspects of the adult personality in both normal and neurotic persons. In neurotics, conflicts arising from unconscious thoughts, in particular thoughts of a sexual nature, produced the neurosis. Thus, in this new formulation, repressed childhood fantasies of seduction took the place of actual childhood seduction as the causative factor in Freud's theory of hysteria.

In *The Interpretation of Dreams* Freud argued these points, using sample dreams to illustrate each of them. He also described the methods by which dream censorship disguised dream content and postulated a model of the mind in which there were unconscious and conscious functional components as well as an intermediate preconscious stage. In the remainder of this chapter we will follow Freud's reasoning as he develops his theory.

Freud begins *The Interpretation of Dreams* by stating:

In the following pages, I shall demonstrate that there is a psychological technique which makes it possible to interpret dreams, and that on the application of this technique, every dream will reveal itself as a psychological structure, full of significance, and one which may be assigned to a specific place in the psychic activities of the waking state. Further, I shall endeavor to elucidate the processes which underlie the strangeness and obscurity of dreams, and to deduce from these processes the nature of the psychic forces whose conflict or cooperation is responsible for our dreams.

After presenting a short historical summary of man's conception of dreaming, Freud discusses a sample dream of his own, his "specimen dream" which he uses to illustrate his theory that every dream is the fulfillment of an unconscious wish. Freud examines this dream in some detail and I wish to do the same. It has become a focus of psychoanalytic interest, and I will be using it in the next chapter to illustrate later developments in psychoanalysis and also in the third section of this book in connection with my own hypotheses concerning the evolutionary origin and meaning of dreams.

Freud's specimen dream occurred in the summer of 1895. He was staying with his wife and family at Schloss Belle Vue, a resort hotel outside Vienna. Freud relates that he had been treating a young woman, Emma, for hysterical anxiety. Emma (called Irma in Freud's presentation of his dream) was a friend of the family and had been recommended to Freud by Josef Breuer. Freud had broken off treatment with Emma for the summer on a discordant note. He had relieved Emma of a number of anxiety symptoms, but she had retained serious somatic problems such as intense retching. Before going on vacation, Freud had suggested a psychological interpretation to Emma that he considered central to her neurosis. Emma refused the interpretation, and Freud was annoyed.

On the day before the dream, Freud was visited by Dr. Oskar Rie, a friend and junior colleague who was the pediatrician to Freud's children. Rie had been staying with Emma and her family in the country and, in answer to Freud's query about Emma's health, had replied that "She is better, but not quite well." Freud was disturbed by this, thinking that Rie might be taking the part of Emma's parents (who disapproved of Freud) against him. Freud was also concerned about his skill in treating Emma and that same evening wrote an extended description of Emma's case to Breuer in order to justify himself. The dream occurred that night and involved five characters, Freud himself, Emma (Irma in Freud's account of the dream), Breuer (called Dr. M.), Rie (called Otto), and another young physician, a colleague of Rie's and Freud's, who appears as Leopold in the dream. The dream was the following:

A great hall—a number of guests, whom we are receiving—among them Irma, whom I immediately take aside, as though to answer her letter, and to reproach her for not yet accepting the "solution." I say to her: "If you still have pains, it is really only your own fault." She answers: "If you only knew what pains I have now in the throat, stomach, and abdomen—I am choked by them." I am startled, and look at her. She looks pale and puffy. I think that after all I must be overlooking some organic affection. I take her to the window and look into her throat. She offers some resistance to this, like a woman who has a set of false teeth. I think, surely, she doesn't need them. The mouth then opens wide, and I find a large white spot on the right, and elsewhere I see extensive gray-ish-white scabs adhering to curiously curled formations, which are evidently shaped like the turbinal bones of the nose—I quickly call Dr. M., who repeats the examination and confirms it. . . . Dr. M. looks quite unlike his usual self; he is very pale, he limps, and his chin is clean-shaven. . . . Now my friend Otto, too, is standing beside her, and my friend Leopold percusses her covered chest, and says: "She has a dullness below, on the left," and also calls attention to an infiltrated portion of skin on the left shoulder (which I can feel, in spite of the dress). . . . M. says: "There's no doubt that it's an infection, but it doesn't matter; dysentery will follow and the poison will be eliminated." . . . We know, too, precisely how the infection originated. My friend Otto, not long ago, gave her, when she was feeling unwell, an injection of a preparation of propyl . . . propyls . . . propionic acid . . . trimethylamin (the formula of which I see before me, printed in heavy type). . . . One doesn't give such injections so rashly. . . . Probably, too, the syringe was not clean.

Freud begins his analysis of this dream with the statement that the dream has an advantage over many others in that its subject matter is clear—it relates to the events of the previous day and to his concern over the treatment of Emma. Freud goes on to say:

Nevertheless . . . I am puzzled by the morbid symptoms of which Irma complains in the dream, for they are not the symptoms for which I treated her. I smile at the nonsensical idea of an injection of proprionic acid and at Dr. M's attempt at consolation. . . . In order to learn the significance of all these details, I resolve to undertake an exhaustive analysis.

Freud then presents his associations to each element of the dream. Freud's associations take him back to his anxieties concerning his medical ability. He feels as though Otto had said to him in the dream: "You do not take your medical duties seriously enough; you are not conscientious; you do not perform what you promise." He is reminded of several similar situations in his medical practice. The scabby turbinal bones in Irma's throat bring him back to his own use of cocaine to suppress swellings in his nose and his recommendation of cocaine to a dear friend (Ernst von Fleischl) who had subsequently died as the result of the use of the drug. He is led to this same thought when he follows his associations to the injection Otto gave to Irma in the dream. He states that he had recommended cocaine to his friend for internal use only to aid in withdrawal from morphine addiction, but that his friend had injected himself with the drug and had died as a consequence.

Freud is reminded of another case in which he prescribed a drug (sulphonal), which was at the time harmless but led to the death of a woman patient. At that time Freud actually turned to Breuer (Dr. M.) for help as he did in the dream. A third case is recalled in association with Dr. M.'s comment "dysentery will follow and the poison will be eliminated." Freud had seen fit not to treat a case he believed to be hysterical dysentery and had sent the young man in question off on a sea voyage. A few days prior to the dream, the young man had written a despairing letter to Freud saying he was ill again. Freud states:

I cannot help reproaching myself for putting the invalid in a position where he might contract some organic affliction of the bowels in addition to his hysteria.

The main message Freud takes from the dream is a condemnation of Otto and a defense of his own conscientiousness. To the element of the dream "One doesn't give such injections so rashly," Freud makes the following association:

Here the reproach of rashness is hurled directly at my friend Otto. I believe I had some such thought in the afternoon, when he seemed to indicate, by word and look, that he had taken sides against me. It was, perhaps: "How easily he is influenced; how irresponsibly he pronounces judgment." Further, the above sentence points once more to my deceased friend, who so irresponsibly resorted to cocaine injections. As I have said I had not intended that injections of the drug should be taken.

And to the dream element "Probably the syringe was not clean" he associates:

Another reproach directed at Otto, but originating elsewhere. On the previous day I happened to meet the son of an old lady of eighty-two, to whom I am obliged to give two injections of morphia daily. At present she is in the country, and I have heard that she is suffering from phlebitis. I immediately thought that this might be a case of infiltration caused by a dirty syringe. It is my pride that in two years I have not given her a single infiltration; I am always careful, of course, to see that the syringe is perfectly clean. For I am conscientious.

Freud sums up his analysis in the words:

For the result of the dream is, that it is not I who am to blame for the pain which Irma is still suffering, but that Otto is to blame for it. Now Otto has annoyed me by his remark about Irma's imperfect cure; the dream avenges me upon him, in that it turns the reproach upon himself. The dream acquits me of responsibility for Irma's condition, as it refers this condition to other causes (which do, indeed, furnish quite a number of explanations). The dream represents a certain state of affairs, such as I might wish to exist; *the content of the dream is thus the fulfilment of a wish; its motive is a wish.*

He closes his discussion of this dream with the following comments:

> I do not wish to assert that I have entirely revealed the meaning of the dream, or that my interpretation is flawless. I could still spend much time upon it; I could draw further explanations from it, and discuss further problems which it seems to propound. I can even perceive the points from which further mental associations might be traced; but such considerations as are always involved in every dream of one's own prevent me from interpreting it farther. Those who are overready to condemn such reserve should make the experiment of trying to be more straightforward. For the present I am content with the one fresh discovery which has just been made: If the method of dream-interpretation here indicated is followed, it will be found that dreams do really possess a meaning, and are by no means the expression of a disintegrated cerebral activity, as the writers on the subject would have us believe. When the work of interpretation has been completed the dream can be recognized as a wish-fulfillment.

Before leaving Freud's analysis of his specimen dream, there are several additional associations we should note. They do not affect Freud's main theme but will be important to us later. Besides Dr. M. (Breuer) there are two young doctors who attend Irma. They are Otto (Oskar Rie) and Leopold. Freud's association to these two men is the following:

> My friend Leopold also is a physician, and a relative of Otto's. Since the two practise the same speciality, fate has made them competitors, so that they are constantly being compared with one another. Both of them assisted me for years, while I was still directing a public clinic for neurotic children. There, scenes like that reproduced in my dream had often taken place. While I

would be discussing the diagnosis of a case with Otto, Leopold would examine the child anew and make an unexpected contribution towards our decision. There was a difference of character between the two men . . . Otto was remarkably prompt and alert; Leopold was slow and thoughtful, but thorough. If I contrast Otto and the cautious Leopold in the dream I do so, apparently, in order to extol Leopold.

To Otto's injection of "a preparation of propyl . . . propyls . . . proprionic acid" Freud makes these comments:

How on earth did this occur to me? During the previous evening before I wrote out the case history and had the dream, my wife opened a bottle of liqueur labelled "Ananas" which was a present from our friend Otto. . . . This liqueur smelt so strongly of fusel oil that I refused to drink it. . . . The smell of fusel oil (amyl) has now apparently awakened my memory of the whole series: propyl, methyl, etc. which furnished the preparation of propyl mentioned in the dream.

To the term "trimethylamin," Freud makes these associations:

In the dream I see the chemical formula of this substance—which at all events is evidence of a great effort on the part of my memory —and the formula is even printed in heavy type, as though to distinguish it from the context as something of particular importance. And where does trimethylamin, thus forced on my attention, lead me? To a conversation with another friend, who for years has been familiar with all my germinating ideas, and I with his [Wilhelm Fliess whom we shall meet later]. . . . At that time he had just informed me of certain ideas concerning a sexual chemistry, and had mentioned, among others, that he thought he had found in trimethylamin one of the products of sexual metabolism. This substance thus leads me to sexuality, the factor to which I attribute the greatest significance in respect to the origin of these nervous affections which I am trying to cure. . . .

I surmise why it is that the formula of trimethylamin is so insistent in the dream. So many important things are centred about this one word: trimethylamin is an allusion, not merely to the all-important factor of sexuality, but also to a friend whose sympathy I remember with satisfaction whenever I feel isolated in my opinions. And this friend, who plays such a large part in my life: will he not appear yet again in the concatenation of ideas peculiar to this dream? Of course; he has a special knowledge of the results of affections of the nose and the sinuses, and has revealed to science several highly remarkable relations between the turbinal bones and the female sexual organs. (The three curly formations in Irma's throat.) I got him to examine Irma, in order to determine whether her gastric pains were of nasal origin. But he himself suffers from suppurative rhinitis, which gives me concern. . . .

Finally, Freud concludes that in the dream he is deriding Breuer. In connection with Dr. M.'s diagnosis that "dysentery will follow," etc. Freud states:

I am making fun of Dr. M., for I recollect that years ago he once jestingly told a very similar story of a colleague. He had been called in to consult with him in the case of a woman who was very seriously ill, and he felt obliged to confront his colleague, who seemed very hopeful, with the fact that he found albumen in the patient's urine. His colleague, however, did not allow this to worry him, but answered calmly: "That does not matter, my dear sir; the albumen will soon be excreted!" Thus I can no longer doubt that this part of the dream expresses derision for those of my colleagues who are ignorant of hysteria. . . . But what can be my motive in treating this friend so badly? That is simple enough: Dr. M. agrees with my solution as little as does Irma herself [presumably Freud's sexual interpretation of the cause of Emma's hysteria]. Thus in the dream I have already revenged myself on two persons: on Irma in the words, "If you still have pains, it is your own fault," and on

Dr. M. in the wording of the nonsensical consolation which has been put into his mouth.

Proceeding from an analysis of the meaning of the Irma dream, Freud takes his first look at the structure of dreams. He uses his specimen dream and others to draw the distinction between the manifest and latent content of a dream. The manifest content is the immediate story related by the dream while the latent content is its underlying meaning—the wish which is disguised by the dream censor before it appears as the manifest content. (For his sample dream, Freud chose one that was relatively straightforward, compared to some, in its manifest content and, on the level that Freud analyzed it, not overly censored.) The concept of day residue is also illustrated by the Irma dream. Freud states that for every dream, a dream stimulus is to be found among the experiences or thoughts of the day preceding the dream. In the case of the Irma dream the stimulus was clearly Oskar Rie's visit to Freud.

I pause here to note that the Irma dream seems to lack some of the essential elements of dreams Freud postulates later in *The Interpretation of Dreams,* namely, a tie to the past and a sexual basis. Freud may have been referring to these matters when he said, "I can even perceive the points from which further mental associations might be traced, but such considerations as are always involved in every dream of one's own prevent me from interpreting it further." In 1954, the psychoanalyst Erik Erikson supplied these missing dimensions in an extensive reexamination of the Irma dream. In this study, Erikson notes that the German word Freud used for "syringe" in the phrase "the syringe was not clean" was *Spritze. Spritze* does indeed mean "syringe" but also has the colloquial meaning of "squirter," which has many connotations. In Erikson's analysis, the relevant one is the allusion to the penis and urinating. The use of a dirty syringe thus makes Otto a "dirty squirter" or a "little squirt" not just a careless physician. Erikson then observes that a little further on in *The Interpretation of Dreams,* Freud reports one of his earliest childhood memories:

Then, when I was seven or eight years of age another domestic incident occurred which I remember very well. One evening before going to bed I had disregarded the dictates of discretion, and had satisfied my needs in my parents' bedroom, and in their presence. Reprimanding me for this delinquency, my father remarked: "That boy will never amount to anything." This must have been a terrible affront to my ambition, but allusions to this scene recur again and again in my dreams, and are constantly coupled with enumerations of my accomplishments and successes, as though I wanted to say: "You see, I have amounted to something after all."

Erikson suggests that this crime and its associated shame became forcefully associated in Freud's mind with his chances of ever becoming a man who amounted to anything—a man who kept his promises. Thus Freud must have been acutely sensitive to implications of the sort Oskar Rie had raised—that he had promised to cure Emma's hysteria and had not. Hence in Freud's dream, Rie (Otto) became the dirty squirter, not Freud. Erikson further suggests that in Freud's unconscious mind, Otto's putting "dirty solution" in the wrong place may have been associated with this childhood act of urination in his parents' bedroom (presumably, Erikson thinks, in a chamber pot) and that further ideas of a sexual nature were also associated in Freud's unconscious mind with this act.

These additional associations may or may not be valid—there is no way of knowing when the meaning of the dream is not being derived from the free associations of the dreamer. However, this is the kind of substrate of the Irma dream that Freud's theory would require.

Following the analysis of his specimen dream, Freud raises the question of the obvious existence of unpleasant dreams, dreams that are seemingly the opposite of wish-fulfilling. He then proceeds to encompass them into his theory by a means that cannot help but make the concept of a wish and who is wishing somewhat unclear. Thus:

In the sexual constitution of many persons there is a masochistic component, which has arisen through the conversion of the aggressive, sadistic component into its opposite. Such people are called "ideal" masochists if they seek pleasure not in the bodily pain which may be inflicted upon them, but in humiliation and psychic chastisement. It is obvious that such persons may have counter-wish-dreams and disagreeable dreams, yet these are for them nothing more than wish-fulfilments, which satisfy their masochistic inclinations.

And later in the book:

But how is it possible for a dream to place itself at the service of self-criticism, and to take as its content a rational warning instead of a prohibited wish-fulfilment? I have already hinted that the answer to this question presents many difficulties. We may conclude that the foundation of the dream consisted at first of an arrogant phantasy of ambition; but that in its stead only its suppression and abasement has reached the dream-content. One must remember that there are masochistic tendencies in mental life to which such an inversion might be attributed.

When in a later theory (our next chapter) Freud partitioned the personality into ego, id, and superego, dreams of this nature, so-called punishment dreams, became wish-fulfilling dreams of the superego.

Freud goes on to consider a number of other issues. He makes the observation that all dreams of a night deal with the same subject matter (he was, of course, unaware of REM sleep and the periodic occurrence of four or five dreams every night). He notes that the subject matter may change from one night to the next or a single concern may capture the attention of dreams for days at a time or longer. By what criteria are the subject matter of dreams selected on a given night? Freud does not deal with this point in depth, but states that there are dreams from above and dreams from below. A dream from below is provoked by a repressed unconscious wish that has found a means of being represented in some of the day's events—these events then appear as the day residues of the manifest dream. A dream from above is initiated by thoughts emanating from daytime activities which continue during the night and manage to obtain reinforcement from an association with an unconscious wish.

Freud asks what is the function of dreams. He does not consider the expression of repressed unconscious wishes in dreams as the function of dreams (such expression does not benefit the individual, for example) but merely as a phenomenon that occurs during the sleeping state. That is, as a result of weakened repression during sleep, unconscious material inevitably surfaces periodically in the form of dreams. It does not appear essential in Freud's theory that he provide a function. However, he does provide one. He postulates that dreams are the guardian of sleep. Without dreams the emergence of repressed thoughts would awaken the sleeper. The dream encapsulates the repressed material and allows its expression without disturbing sleep.

Although Freud does not discuss the factors that determine the choice of one subject matter over another for a given night's dreaming, he notes that the subject matter of all dreams has a common characteristic. It is all psychically significant—there are no trivial dreams. And the latent content of dreams carries the "mark of the beast"—the unconscious wishes of an immoral, incestuous, or otherwise perverse nature. As an example, Freud considers the question of sibling rivalry.

Freud observes that the child of three or four years of age is absolutely egotistical—it feels its needs acutely and strives remorselessly to satisfy them. Freud cites children wanting the stork to take an infant brother or sister back whence it came, and an instance of a three-year-old little girl trying to strangle an infant sibling in its cradle. He goes on to say that he has found dreams of the death of brothers and sisters, denoting intense hostility, in all of his female patients. This dream content, derived from the analysis of adult dreams, presumably reflected childhood wishes repressed in the unconscious. One patient remembered as an adult a dream she had at the age of four: "A number of children, all of her brothers and sisters with her boy and girl cousins, were romping about in a meadow. Suddenly they all grew wings, flew up, and were gone." Freud notes that this child at the age of four, upon asking what happens to children when they die, may have been told by an adult that they become angels, grow wings, and fly away. In the dream, the child expressed the wish that her siblings and cousins, seen as her competitors, do just that.

In mitigation of these seemingly horrendous childhood wishes, Freud points out that death means something quite different to a child than to an adult:

> But how does the childish character arrive at such heights of wickedness as to desire the death of a rival or a stronger playmate, as though all misdeeds could be atoned for only by death? Those who speak in this fashion forget that the child's idea of "being dead" has little but the word in common with our own. The child knows nothing of the horrors of decay, of shivering in the cold grave, of the terror of the infinite Nothing, the thought of which the adult, as all the myths of the hereafter testify, finds so intolerable. The fear of death is alien to the child; and so he plays with the horrid word, and threatens another child: "If you do that again, you will die, just like Francis died"; at which the poor mother shudders, unable perhaps to forget that the greater proportion of mortals do not survive beyond the years of childhood. Even at the age of eight, a child returning from a visit to a natural history museum may say to her mother: "Mamma, I do love you so; if you ever die, I am going to have you stuffed and set you up here in the room, so that I can always, always see you!" So different from our own is the childish conception of being dead.

Freud then turns to the Oedipus complex, the childhood wish of the little boy for the death of his father, and its counterpart on the female side, the Electra complex. He notes once again that these wishes are found in his patient's dreams and states his belief that they are present in the unconscious minds of normal people as well. (One assumes that Freud's dreams revealed this wish in his own unconscious mind.) Freud cites the common experience of the little boy, having been allowed to sleep with Mommy while Daddy is away on a trip saying that it would be nice if Daddy continued to be absent. Or the little girl saying, "Now Mommy can go away and then I can be Daddy's wife." He further remarks on the common tendency of mothers to dote on their sons while fathers dote on their daughters, and the child's natural reaction toward the parent of the same sex when that parent might want to oppose the relationship. As an example of a case of neurosis caused by a repressed wish for the death of a parent, Freud gives the following history:

> I had the opportunity of obtaining a profound insight into the unconscious psychic life of a young man for whom an obsessional neurosis made life almost unendurable, so that he could not go into the streets, because he was tormented by the fear that he would kill everyone he met. He spent his days contriving evidence of an alibi in case he should be accused of any murder that might have been committed in the city. It goes without saying that this man was as moral as he was highly cultured. The analysis—which, by the way, led to a cure—revealed, as the basis of this distressing obsession, murderous impulses in respect of his rather overstrict father—impulses which, to his astonishment, had consciously expressed themselves when he was seven years old, but which, of course, had originated in a much earlier period of his childhood. After the painful illness and death of his father, when the young man was in his thirty-first year, the obsessive reproach made its appearance, which transferred itself to strangers in the form of this phobia. Anyone capable of wishing to push his own father from a mountain top into an abyss cannot be trusted to spare the lives of persons less closely related to him; he therefore does well to lock himself into his room.

Freud adds the final dimension to the Oedipal drama by contending that the young boy wants to possess his mother sexually over and above wanting her exclusive love and attention. Freud bases this view again on relatively transparent as well as disguised occurrences of this fantasy in dreams. The ability to conceive this fantasy on the part of the little boy is presumably based in childhood observation of acts of sexual intercourse. I will return to this most controversial aspect of Freud's theory in a later chapter of this book.

That the latent content of dreams should contain childhood murderous wishes may not be so surprising in the light of Freud's explanation. These wishes are not judged as being horrible when expressed by children (hostility toward siblings is merely naughty and should be corrected) but acquire their shocking characteristics when, as Freud suggests, they are retained in the adult unconscious. Another type of unconscious wish arising in the adult mind strikes one as decidedly more perverse. In an addition to *The Interpretation of Dreams* made after the First World War, Freud relates a dream of his own that concerns his son Martin, who was in active service on the German side in that war. He dreams that fellow officers of his son's unit send a sum of money and a citation, an honorable mention, to Freud. Freud's son appears before him, not in a military uniform but in a tight-fitting sports outfit and a cap, and proceeds to climb up on a basket near a chest to put something in the chest. His son's face is bandaged. Freud wonders if his son has false teeth. Freud wakes up at 2:30 in the morning, without anxiety but with heart palpitations.

Freud's associations to this dream lead him to the imagined death of his son in combat. The money and the honorable mention have been sent back by fellow officers because of this. The sports outfit his son is wearing makes him look like a child, and Freud remembers an incident in which Freud himself, as a child, reached up on a chest, slipped, and knocked his jaw on the chest with sufficient force so that his teeth might have been knocked out. Freud comments:

> At this point, an admonition [to his son] presents itself: it serves you right—like a hostile impulse against the valiant warrior. A profounder analysis enables me to detect the hidden impulse, which would be able to find satisfaction in the dreaded mishap to my son. It is the envy of youth which the elderly man [Freud was about sixty] believes that he has thoroughly stifled in actual life.

There is every indication that Freud was a loving father, and yet this wish for his son's death is in his unconscious mind. Dreams in which a father, thoroughly moral and not overly lustful, finds himself having sexual intercourse with his daughter, fall into the same category. Freud points out that dreams frequently contain wishes on a second level, later in origin than early childhood wishes. In the Irma dream for example, the wish on the adult level was that Freud be exonerated for responsibility in the treatment of Irma. Using Erikson's interpretation, this would be associated with the childhood memory of urinating in his parents' bedroom and its ultimate source might be an Oedipal fantasy the young Freud harbored as he displayed himself in that situation. Freud's wish that his son die arose in his unconscious mind as an adult. According to Freud, there was an associated childhood incident and presumably a childhood fantasy from which the adult wish arose. The point to be made is that, in Freud's view, repressed ideas of early childhood maintain their influence and may form the basis of later unconscious fantasies or wishes of a bizarre and wholly immoral character.

Leaving the question of dream content, Freud, in the remainder of *The Interpretation of Dreams*, explores the means the dream censor uses to disguise dream content and constructs a model of the organization of the mind. I will now summarize these ideas. For our later analysis we must bear in mind that the mechanisms that Freud describes as dream distortions and disguise by a censor, whether they be censorship or not, must be addressed by any theory that seeks to explain dreams.

Freud delineates four mechanisms of dream distortion and censorship—condensation, displacement, representability, and symbolism—which together disguise the latent content of a dream and are responsible for the bizarre quality of the dream. In discussing condensation, Freud observes that the story told by the dream—its manifest content —is much more succinct than the associations that the dreamer makes to this material. He cites the amount of space he requires to write a dream down as compared to writing out its associations. (For example, in the Irma dream Freud's statement of the dream occupied half a page in *The Interpretation of Dreams* while its associations took almost eight pages—I presented only some of them in this chapter.) The condensation does not necessarily occur when one compares a statement of the latent content with its manifest content. Thus Freud's wish that he not be held responsible for Irma's condition—the latent content of the Irma dream—can be stated fully in a few sentences. Condensation takes place only when one compares all of the associations to the elements of the dream with the dream itself—thus the term "condensation" is derived from Freud's concept that all of these associations are represented in condensed form in the dream. Freud goes on to say that condensation is responsible in part for the disconnected quality of some dreams, for they are condensed packets arising from somewhat disparate though related dream-thoughts, pieced together to tell the story of the dream.

Another form of condensation contributing to the bizarre aspect of dreams is the formation of composite figures—actors in the dream who simultaneously represent two or more people. There is an example in the Irma dream. Freud had noted in the course of his associations to that dream that Dr. M. (Breuer) was pale, walked with a limp, and was clean shaven. Breuer was in reality pale but did not have a limp and wore a beard. Freud's associations led him to his older half brother living in England* who was clean shaven and did, because of a recent arthritic condition, walk with a limp. In Freud's view, Dr. M. in the dream represented a fusion of the two men. The reason for the fusion was that in Freud's unconscious mind the two men were in a common category—he was on bad terms with both of them for each had rejected a certain proposal he had made. The proposal to his brother was not specified, but in the case of Breuer the proposal might have been Freud's sexual interpretation of Irma's hysteria, or an issue related to Freud's disagreement with Breuer concerning the theory of the etiology of hysteria.

Freud goes on to give examples of a third form of condensation—the formation of contracted words which represent several ideas simultaneously. One example is the dream of a patient in which a signboard reading "unclamparra" refers to malaria, the disease that she was thought to have but did not (the symptoms were hysterical) and eucalyptus, trees planted to dry up the swampland near a monastery she had visited. Eucalyptus and malaria were combined into "unclamparra." Also the patient had drunk a liqueur at the monastery made of eucalyptus. Drinking reminded her of her recent betrothal to a man named Dry, which had broken up over the issue of his drunkenness. In all, a large body of psychologically significant information was condensed in this composite word.

The major conclusion drawn by Freud regarding condensation concerns the relationship between the manifest dream, the associations to the dream, and the dream's latent content. Starting from an element of the manifest dream, associations do not lead directly back to an element of the latent content which represents its underlying meaning; rather each element of the manifest content leads to branching associations which diverge. (One can conceive of this as happening in a downward direction, from manifest toward latent content.) Branches from a given element of the manifest dream may meet again lower in the associative tree, or they may not. The structure of the associations is the same as described by Freud in his lecture on the etiology of hysteria for tracing the memory of a trauma back to memories in earlier life. Ultimately, a given element of the manifest dream may be traced to one or more than one element of the latent content, and in the process, smaller subplots may be revealed. As an example of an element of the manifest dream relating to more than one element of the latent content, Freud takes Dr. M.'s statement "dysentery will follow and the poison will be eliminated" in the Irma dream. To the word "dysentery" Freud associates the word "diphtheria" which he states sounds not unlike "dysentery." (The words in German are *Diphtherie* and *Dysenterie.)* "Diphtheria" leads to the further association that this disease may be the source of the general infection diagnosed by Leopold, the large white spot in Irma's throat being a symptom of the disease. Finally this line of association in the downward direction leads to one part of the latent content—the part that says to Freud, "Irma's illness is organic, not mental." On the other hand, the word "dysentery" also reminds Freud of the young man suffering from hysterical dysentery that he sent on a sea voyage, an act that he does feel may have been negligent. This association leads to a second element of the latent wish, the part that denies wrongdoing and says, "I am not a negligent physician." A subplot of this chain of association is that Dr. M. (Breuer) reminds Freud of his older brother. He dislikes both of them for opposing him and classes them together.

The analysis of this dream has been pursued in the downward direction, from manifest to latent content. This is the direction taken by psychoanalysis in which the subject attempts to free associate to elements of the manifest dream. As I mentioned, in *The Interpretation of Dreams*, Freud conceives of dreams as being initiated from above (events of the day) or below (an unconscious wish), but if the dream is initiated from above it must first become associated with an unconscious wish before the material can be expressed in a dream. In either case, Freud views dreams as constructed in the upward direction, from latent wish to manifest dream. Looking at the example from Irma's dream in this direction, one sees that the two elements of the latent wish—"Irma's illness is organic, not mental" and "I am not a negligent physician"—have converged via "diphtheria" and "the patient that went on a sea voyage" onto the single concept of dysentery. Freud calls this convergence onto a single element of the manifest dream overdetermination. He states that it seems to him that the manifest dream is constructed on the basis of the strength of such convergence—those elements that are the most overdetermined get to constitute the manifest dream.

After considering condensation, Freud turns to the second mechanism of dream censorship, displacement. Freud refers to dreams in which, starting from a manifest dream that seems trivial, one finds, on tracing back through the associated dream-thought, a body of thought that is psychologically significant and charged with emotion. Freud claims that in such dreams the psychological intensity has been displaced from significant to insignificant material, since this was the only way that the emotionally charged ideas of the latent wish in the unconscious mind could evade the censor and gain representation in the dream. As an example, Freud cites his own dream of merely seeing a book, a botanical monograph with colored plates, in a bookseller's window. The chain of association leads to a theme of considerable emotional impact similar to that of the Irma dream, namely his self-justification as a serious medical scholar. Freud states that displacement is the most essential work of the censor, but admits that such displacement is not present in all dreams. The Irma dream, with a clear link in content and emotion between manifest and latent components of the dream, serves as an example of a dream without displacement.

Freud now considers the question he calls representability. The major point is that words or abstract ideas cannot be represented as themselves—the dream must portray them as visual images. As a present-day example, a young man might be attracted to a girl but fearful of involvement, having been romantically hurt before. His unconscious thought might be that the girl could get under his skin and break his heart. The idea appears in his dream as an episode in which a splinter, double pronged somewhat in the shape of the crotch of a tree, has gotten through his skin, is traveling through his bloodstream, and may pierce his heart. Freud gives a rather nice example of a dream image representing an abstract idea:

> There is a terrible storm outside; a miserable hotel—the water is dripping from the walls, and the beds are damp.

The abstract idea is the word "superfluous," which the unconscious mind arrives at via the way station "superfluid."

Freud notes the frequent occurrence of puns and the exchange of similar-sounding words in dreams. As a result, the unconscious mind gains the reputation of being quite witty. An example would be dreaming of a female horse, a mare, which turns out via a number of associations to represent mère, or the dreamer's mother. Finally, Freud states that when spoken utterances do appear in dreams they invariably represent a speech remembered from daytime activity.

The last mechanism of censorship that Freud discusses is perhaps the most well known: the use of symbols to represent genital organs and sexual acts in dreams. Freud finds that in their dreams his patients commonly use elongated objects to represent a penis—for example, sticks, tree trunks, umbrellas (on account of their opening which may be likened to an erection), and guns. (An American folk song satirizes the seemingly all-embracing nature of these symbols with the comment that to psychoanalysts, a penis is anything taller than it is wide.) Similarly, small boxes, chests, cupboards, ovens, cavities, ships, and all kinds of vessels are used to represent the vagina, while steep inclines, ladders, or stairs going up or down are symbolic representations of sexual intercourse. Freud was aware of the danger of easy and loose interpretation of symbols. This was compounded by his finding that free association frequently stops short of a definitive clue as to what the symbol really represents in the dream. In *The Interpretation of Dreams* he recommends careful study of the symbols in especially transparent dreams where the meaning of the symbol can be ascertained in order to "silence the reproach of arbitrariness in dream interpretation." As an example of an instance in which the meaning of a symbol was clear, Freud cites a dream of a patient he was treating for fear of leaving home (agoraphobia).

> I am walking in the street in summer; I am wearing a straw hat of peculiar shape, the middle piece of which is bent upwards, while the side pieces hang downwards (here the description hesitates), and in such a fashion that one hangs lower than the other. I am cheerful and in a confident mood, and as I pass a number of young officers, I think to myself: you can't do anything to me.

Freud relates that the patient could produce no association to the dream so he offered the interpretation that the hat represented a male genital organ, the raised middle with the two downward hanging side pieces. He did not comment on the unequal hanging of the side pieces. Freud wondered at the oddity of the patient's dream using a hat to represent part of a man but recollected that "getting under the cap" was an idiomatic expression for getting married. In previous sessions, Freud had suggested to the patient that her agoraphobia was a reaction to her anxiety over her unconscious sexual-temptation fantasies—and that the meaning of the present dream was that having a husband with such splendid genitals, she would not have to fear the officers.

Freud reports that on hearing the interpretation, the patient withdrew the description of the hat and would not admit that the two side pieces hung down. However, Freud was certain that he had heard the description and insisted she had given it. She was quiet for a while, and then found the courage to ask why it was that one of her husband's testicles was lower than the other and was it the same with all men. With this explained, the patient accepted the interpretation.

Freud views symbolism as another example of censorship, whereby as a result of the disguise offered by the symbol, sexual material is allowed to enter the manifest content of the dream. With the definition and illustration of the four sources of dream distortion, condensation, displacement, representability, and symbolism, Freud proceeds to the last task of his book, the formulation of a theory of the organization of the mind.

In Freud's model, the body of infantile and early childhood memories, fantasies, and thoughts constitute the lowest stratum of the unconscious mind. Herein lie the Oedipal fantasies and similar ideas unacceptable to the conscious mind. These thoughts are repressed but are constantly seeking expression. Fantasies and ideas derived from this early childhood constellation, but referring to events later in life (like Freud's wish that his son die) are also repressed in the unconscious. During sleep, the repression is somewhat relaxed, and the unconscious wishes do manage to express themselves in dreams. But repression is not totally relaxed—a censor in the unconscious (the source of the repression) disguises the unconscious material before it is allowed to find expression in the manifest dream. The censor utilizes condensation, displacement, the need for representability, and symbolization for this purpose.

The disguised wishes do not yet penetrate upward into the manifest dream to be remembered consciously in the morning. There is a sublayer below consciousness called the preconscious. The thought content of the preconscious is similar to that of the conscious except that thoughts in the preconscious are not being attended to at a given moment. For example, the recollection of the name of a person one may have met a day or so ago may not be present in one's consciousness at a given moment, but that recollection is not repressed in the unconscious—it is present in the preconscious and may be recalled by directing conscious attention to the past meeting. According to Freud, the preconscious thinks rationally just as does the conscious and attempts to organize thoughts in an orderly manner. It plays a part in forming the manifest dream in that, when the disguised elements of the unconscious wish rise to the preconscious level, this agency of the mind organizes them as best it can into a coherent story. Freud calls this process of organization of the dream secondary elaboration. Freud also alludes to possible censorship under certain circumstances between the preconscious and conscious, but this is not a major aspect of his model.

How does this mental organization all come about? Freud offers a developmental explanation. It starts with the infant faced with great physical needs. The infant has been fed and thus has had an experience of satisfaction, but now grows hungry anew and cries or struggles help-lessly. As a result of the earlier experience, there is an association of hunger with the memory of being fed, and a psychic need to revive the memory occurs—a wish for satisfaction. In this situation, the child revives the perception of being fed, and this constitutes the wish fulfill-ment. Freud suggests that the infant may actually hallucinate the wished-for bottle or breast. Thus "We may assume a primitive state of the psychic apparatus in which this path is actually followed, i.e., in which the wish ends in hallucination."

Freud states that this mode of psychic functioning is superseded by action to acquire a desired objective in the adult, but it is maintained in its infantile state during dreaming. This is the reason, Freud believes, that almost all dream material is visual. In sleep, action is suppressed. (As we have seen in Chapter 2, motor centers are inhibited during REM sleep.) The wish in the adult unconscious strives for expression in action but is turned back by repression before reaching the conscious level from which action emanates, and is then reflected on an infantile (regressive) path toward hallucination (the dream).

With this model of the mind in place, Freud returns to waking behavior in his neurotic patients and in normal individuals. Freud views neurosis as a result of conflicts arising in the unconscious. The case of the young man suffering from an obsessional neurosis has been cited. In the case of the young woman suffering from agoraphobia, she has an unconscious wish to be seduced by some attractive man she might meet. This wish is reprehensible and is therefore repressed, but as a result of this unconscious wish she suffers so much anxiety whenever she goes out that she confines herself to her home. In her dream, she solves her problem by going out under the protection of her husband's genitals.

In the case of hysteria, Freud postulates a somewhat more compli-

ILLUSTRATION 10

In The Interpretation of Dreams *Freud related the dream to the organization of the mind. There were three levels of organization of the mind, the deepest being the unconscious—above it the preconscious and conscious (shown on the left). The structure of the dream is depicted on the right. Motive power for the dream lay in the unconscious. The dream could emanate from there (dreams from below) or could be stimulated by events in the life of the dreamer that formed an association with an unconscious memory, fantasy, or thought (dreams from above). The latent content of the dream was the unconscious wish, repressed during waking hours but expressed during sleep in the dream. Although repression was relaxed during sleep, it was not absent; a censor in the unconscious distorted and thus disguised dream content. In disguised form, dream thoughts reached the preconscious, where, via secondary elaboration, they were organized into a more coherent (but still characteristically bizarre) manifest dream which could be recalled consciously.*

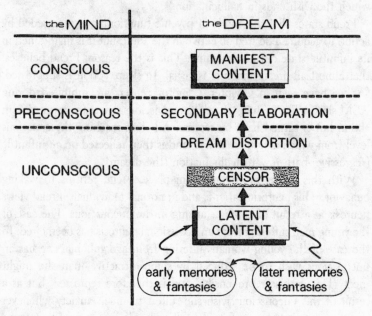

cated mechanism. The hysteric chooses a symptom that at the same time satisfies his or her unconscious wish and serves as a punishment for that wish. Freud offers the example of a female patient with the hysterical symptom of vomiting. The symptom proved to be, on the one hand, the fulfillment of an unconscious fantasy to be continually pregnant—and be made so by as many men as possible—and, on the other, a defensive reaction in that by vomiting she would spoil her figure and beauty and thus no longer be attractive to any man.

Looking beyond neuroses, Freud suggests that unconscious factors have an overriding influence on certain aspects of normal personality such as sexual orientation. As noted, Freud held that the Oedipus complex was universally present in men. Accompanying the desires of the young boy to possess his mother and eliminate his father is a fear of being castrated by his father in retaliation. The boy's unconscious reaction to this fear largely determined his sexuality. Homosexuality of the passive type represents, in the unconscious, a complete surrender to the father to avoid castration. Freud holds that a degree of unconscious homosexuality is present in all men. According to Freudian theory, Oedipal conflicts determine other aspects of behavior besides sex. A present-day Freudian psychoanalyst treating a patient who has only, say, to carry out a trivial step in order to achieve a higher academic degree but refuses, without rational reason, to do so, expects to find a fear of surpassing father in his patient's unconscious. As we shall see, later psychoanalysts, via ego psychology, studied the unconscious underpinnings of the entire personality.

Freud saw the function of psychoanalysis as bringing the unconscious under the domination of the preconscious. And he viewed the analysis of dreams as the royal road to a knowledge of the unconscious. In a later chapter, I will discuss the present-day complexities and difficulties of achieving this objective.

We have now completed a statement of what Freud considered "the most valuable of all the discoveries it has been my good fortune to make." It is a somewhat complicated construction, but Freud has put it in comprehensible if not precise terms. This is the material we will consider in the last section of this book. It will be my view that Freud, in the discovery of free association, the analysis of the structure of dreams, and the elucidation of the unconscious made a momentous contribution to human knowledge. However, I believe that neuroscientific findings suggest an organization of the unconscious mind different from the one he set forth.

To close this chapter we turn to an amazing episode in Freud's life which leads us on a path of inquiry that will be completed only after I have presented my own theory of unconscious organization. The episode was the following: In 1887 Freud met Wilhelm Fliess, a Berlin physician of his own age. Fliess, a nose and throat specialist, had, on the advice of Breuer, attended a lecture Freud gave at the University of Vienna that year. The two men became very close friends and remained so until 1900. Freud and Fliess met periodically at various cities at what they called congresses to discuss personal and scientific ideas. Freud was developing his scientific theories and discussed them in detail with Fliess. Fliess for his part shared Freud's view that the explanation of psychological phenomena would ultimately be found in physiology and was developing several theories of his own. One theory held that the nose influenced a major part of human physiology. There was a "reflex neurosis" arising from the nose which affected the muscles, heart, stomach, and organs of reproduction—the nose was especially connected to the genitals. Another theory held that the twenty-eight-day menstrual period of the female and a presumed twenty-three-day periodicity in the male combined to explain sexuality in men and women and periodic cycles in all living things. Despite the outlandish nature of these ideas, Freud took them seriously and considered Fliess a brilliant physician.

During the course of their friendship, Freud and Fliess exchanged several hundred letters. In these letters Freud wrote to Fliess about the vicissitudes of his life and career and sent Fliess preliminary drafts of his works for criticism. The text of Freud's unpublished "Project for a Scientific Psychology" is available today only because it formed a part of this correspondence. Only Freud's letters to Fliess exist today—the other side of the correspondence was destroyed by Freud. Freud tried to procure his letters to Fliess after Fliess's death, but they were obtained by Princess Marie Bonaparte, a friend and pupil of Freud's, and in 1950 certain of the letters were published under the auspices of a committee of Freud's followers, including his daughter Anna. The remaining correspondence was donated to the Library of Congress with the proviso that they not be revealed until the year 2000. In certain cases, however, individuals have been allowed to read the unpublished material.

In 1966, the psychoanalyst Dr. Max Schur wrote a paper entitled "Some Additional Day Residues of the Specimen Dream of Psychoanalysis" based on his reading of Freud's unpublished letters to Fliess. The letters reveal that in late February of 1895, several months prior to the Irma dream (July 23, 1895) Freud had asked Fliess to come to Vienna to examine his patient Emma (Irma) to see if her somatic symptoms were nasal in origin. Fliess recommended and carried out surgery on Emma's turbinate bone and sinuses and then returned to Berlin several days later. In a letter to Fliess written on March 4, 1895, Freud reports a problem:

Dearest Wilhelm,
    We really can't be satisfied with Emma's condition; persistent swelling, going up and down "like an avalanche," pain to the point where morphine is indispensable, poor nights. The purulent secretion has somewhat decreased since yesterday. The day before yesterday she had a massive hemorrhage, probably because a bone chip the size of a penny had come loose; there were about two bowlfuls. Today we encountered some resistance on irrigation, and because the pain and edema had increased, I let myself be persuaded to call in G. [Gersuny, a prominent Viennese surgeon].
. . . He stated that the access [to the cavity] had considerably contracted and was insufficient for drainage. He inserted a rubber tube and threatened to break it [the bone] open if this didn't stay in. To judge by the smell, all this is probably right. Please send me your authoritative advice. I don't look forward to new surgery on this girl. . . .

The next development was reported in Freud's letter of March 8:

March 8, 1895

Dearest Wilhelm,

Just received your letter and am able to answer it immediately. Fortunately I am finally seeing my way clear and feel reassured about Miss Emma, about whom I can give you a report which will probably upset you as much as me; but I hope you will get over it as fast I have.

I wrote you that the swelling and bleeding wouldn't let up and that suddenly a foetid odor set in along with an obstacle to irrigation (or was the latter new?). I arranged for Gersuny to be called in, and he inserted a drain, hoping that things would work out if discharge were reestablished. Otherwise he behaved in a rather rejecting way. Two days later I was awakened early in the morning —quite profuse bleeding had started again, with pain, etc. I got a telephone message from G[ersuny] that he could come only in the evening, so I asked R (a nose and throat specialist) to meet me (at Miss Emma's apartment). This we did at noon. There was moderate bleeding from the nose and mouth; the foetid odor was very bad. R. cleaned the area surrounding the opening, removed some blood clots which were sticking to the surface, and suddenly pulled at something like a thread. He kept right on pulling, and before either of us had time to think, at least half a meter of gauze had been removed from the cavity. The next moment came a flood of blood. The patient turned white, her eyes bulged, and her pulse was no longer palpable. However, immediately after this he packed the cavity with fresh iodoform gauze, and the hemorrhage stopped. It had lasted about half a minute, but this was enough to make the poor creature, who by then we had lying quite flat, unrecognizable. In the meantime, or actually afterward, something else happened. At the moment the foreign body came out, and everything had become obvious to me, immediately after which I was confronted with the sight of the patient, I felt sick. . . .

I don't think I had been overwhelmed by the blood; affects were welling up in me at that moment. So we had done her an injustice. She had not been abnormal at all, but a piece of iodo-form gauze had gotten torn off when you removed the rest, and stayed in for fourteen days, interfering with the healing process, after which it had torn away and provoked the bleeding. The fact that this mishap should have happened to you, how you would react to it when you learned about it, what others would make of it, how wrong I had been to press you to operate in a foreign city where you couldn't handle the aftercare, how my intention of getting the best for the poor girl was insidiously thwarted, with the resultant danger to her life—all this came over me simultaneously. I have worked it off by now, I was not sufficiently clear headed to think of reproaching R. at that moment. That occurred to me ten minutes later; he should have thought immediately: "There is something there; don't pull it out or you'll start a hemorrhage; stick some more in, take her to Loew and do the cleaning and widening [of the opening to the cavity—obviously the sinus] at the same time." But he was just as surprised as I was.

Now that I have assimilated all this, nothing remains but sincere compassion for my "child of sorrow" *[Schmerzenskind]*. Indeed, I shouldn't have tortured you, but I had every reason to entrust you with such a matter and with even more than this. You handled it as well as possible. The tearing off of the iodoform gauze was one of those accidents that happen to the most fortunate and cautious of surgeons. . . . G[ersuny] mentioned that he had had a similar experience, and that he therefore used iodoform wicks instead of gauze (you must remember this from your own case). Of course no one blames you in any way, nor do I know why they should. And I only hope that you will come as quickly as I did to feel only pity. Rest assured that I felt no need to restore my trust in you. I only want to add that I hesitated for a day to tell you all about it, and that then I began to be ashamed, and here is the letter.

Indeed a startling set of affairs was unfolding. Fliess had committed an unpardonable surgical blunder, and Freud could not wait to place the

blame on the surgeon R. who had helped save Emma's life. The incident was not yet over. On March 28 Freud wrote:

> Dearest Wilhelm,
>   I know what you want to hear first: she is doing tolerably well
> completely calmed down, no fever, no hemorrhage. The packing
> which was inserted six days ago is still in, and we hope to be safe
> from new surprises. Of course, she is starting to develop new hys-
> terias from this past period, which then are being dissolved by me.
>   I must take it in my stride that you are not quite so well either.
> I hope this won't be for long. I suppose you will work your way out
> of it pretty soon. . . .
>   My own condition is not especially bad, but keeps me out of
> sorts. A pulse as irregular as that seems after all to preclude well-
> being.

And in a passage that indicates his unusual emotional attachment to
Fliess, Freud writes:

> In general I miss you badly. Am I really the same person who was
> overflowing with ideas and projects as long as you were within
> reach? When I sit down at my desk in the evening, I often don't
> know what I should work on.

> She, Miss Emma, is doing well; she is a nice, decent girl who does
> not blame either of us in this affair, and who speaks of you with
> high esteem.

> Keep quite well; give me detailed reports about yourself and don't
> take me to task this time. Another time I'll swamp you with letters
> and enclosures. You are steady; I am not.

Two weeks later there was a turn for the worse. On April 11, Freud
wrote:

> Dearest Wilhelm,
>   Gloomy times, unbelievably gloomy. Mainly this business with

Emma which is rapidly deteriorating. I reported to you last time
that G. had inspected the cavity under general anesthesia, pal-
pated it, and declared it satisfactory. We indulged our hopes and
the patient was gradually recovering. However, eight days ago she
began to bleed with the packing in place, something which had
not happened before. She was packed again. The bleeding was
minimal. Two days ago a new hemorrhage, again with the packing
in place, and by now more than ample. New packing, renewed
helplessness. Yesterday, R. wanted to reexamine the cavity. A new
hypothesis about the source of the hemorrhage after the first operation (the one performed by you) had by chance been suggested
by Weil [another surgeon]. As soon as the packing was partly out,
there was a new, highly dangerous hemorrhage, which I witnessed.
It didn't spurt, but it surged, something like a [fluid] level rising
exceedingly fast and then overflowing everything. It must have
been a large vessel; but which one, and where? We of course
couldn't see anything and were glad that the packing was inside
again. Add to this the pain, the morphine, the demoralization
resulting from the obvious medical helplessness, and the whole air
of danger, and you can picture the state the poor girl is in. We
don't know what can be done. R. has been resisting the suggestion
that he perform a ligation of the carotid artery. The danger that
she will start to run a fever is also not far off. I'm really quite
shaken that such a misfortune can have arisen from this operation,
which was depicted as harmless.

This last phrase was the first indication that Freud might blame Fliess
for his error. The specialist Weil was critical of Fliess for his surgery,
and Freud remarked mildly that the operation "was depicted as harmless." The result (incredibly) was a demand by Fliess for vindication.
He expected some sort of testimonial from the surgeon Gersuny that
Gersuny did not share Weil's opinion. Freud wrote back on April 20:

Dearest Wilhelm,
    Of course I immediately informed R. of your suggestions con-
cerning Emma. Naturally things look different from close up, for

example, the hemorrhage. I can assure you that for the surgeons to sit around and wait would have been out of the question. It was bleeding as though from the carotid artery. Within half a minute she would have bled to death. However, she is doing better now. The packing was carefully and gradually removed. There was no mishap, and she is now in the clear.

The writer of this is still very miserable, but is also quite offended that you should deem it necessary to have a testimonial from G. for your rehabilitation. Even if G. should have the same opinion of your skill as Weil, for me you remain the healer, the prototype of the man into whose hands one confidently entrusts one's life and that of one's family. I wanted to tell you of my misery, perhaps ask you for some advice about Emma, but not reproach you for anything. This would have been stupid, unjustified, in clear contradiction to my feelings. . . .

A year later in a letter written to Fliess on April 26, 1896, Freud referred to Emma again.

With regard to Emma, I shall be able to prove to you that you were right; her hemorrhages were hysterical, brought on by longing, probably at the "sexual period." . . .

The entire incident of the iodoform gauze was forgotten. The cause of Emma's bleeding had been shifted to hysteria.

Schur asks the obvious question: How, in his exhaustive analysis of the Irma dream, could Freud not have brought up an association to this traumatic episode? As the reader will recall, associations to Fliess were forthcoming in connection with the word "trimethylamin," which appeared printed in heavy type in the dream. But the associations were innocuous and complimentary, and Emma's operation was skipped over. (Freud's associations to "trimethylamin" are given on page 99.)

Schur considers the possibility that Freud made the association to the traumatic episode and then deliberately withheld it in discussing the dream, but he rejects the idea. It seems to fly in the face of Freud's honesty, and indeed why would Freud have involved himself in a situation of this sort when he could just as easily have chosen another sample dream without this complication. Schur suggests that the episode of Emma's operation did not appear in Freud's associations because it was repressed and that Freud was not thorough enough in his self-analysis to uncover it. Further, Schur observes that had it been uncovered it would have revealed to Freud that the latent wish of the dream was not only to take blame from himself and place it on Otto (who gave a dirty injection) but also to take blame from Fliess and place it on Otto. Thus:

> But it was not only his own exculpation that he [Freud] achieved; it was the need to exculpate Fliess from responsibility for Emma's nearly fatal complications that was probably the strongest (immediate) motive for the constellation of the dream.

Schur asks why this was so and concludes that it resulted from Freud's emotionally dependent reliance on Fliess—an example of transference, a relationship that occurs between a patient under psychoanalysis and his analyst. (The possibility does exist, nonetheless, that Freud did find the Irma dream the ideal specimen dream, and, convinced of his interpretation, did deliberately fail to set down his association to Fliess's surgical error, since the incident was embarrassing to Fliess, and Freud believed it to be unimportant in the interpretation. Freud, in his closing comments on the Irma dream, page 97, did state that he had taken the liberty of withholding certain further associations of a personal nature.)

Whether Schur's explanation is correct or not, his revelations transform Freud's specimen dream of psychoanalysis from an elucidating demonstration of dream analysis to an example of the difficulties involved in dream interpretation. In conjunction with my own hypothesis in the third section of this book, we will find that the Irma dream and Freud's lapse may be explained differently.

The Interpretation of Dreams was just the first step. Freud revised his theories considerably in the years that followed. In addition, other men and women, drawn into the practice of psychoanalysis by Freud's discoveries, made their own observations and formulated their own theories of psychic function. We must consider certain of these later developments in order to establish a proper basis in psychology for later comparison with the findings of neuroscience.

Five

LATER DEVELOPMENTS

In the half-century following *The Interpretation of Dreams*, psychoanalysis, led for the better part of that time by Freud himself, grew into a worldwide movement. It became not only the dominant influence in psychiatry but, via its incorporation into literature, drama, and other parts of our culture, changed the way Western man thought about himself. (This was followed by a decline in its popularity, which I will relate presently, but for now we consider its ascendency.)

We shall see three aspects of psychoanalysis interwoven in its history —first, a body of theory mainly written by Freud himself, second, a method of investigation and therapy that changed over time in its emphasis and the type of person to whom it was applied, and third, an organization, an international association of psychoanalysts allied with Freud with its own strict rules of membership, psychoanalytic journals, and official doctrine. As we follow these developments, we will find that certain psychological phenomena consistently appear and may be taken as our psychoanalytic data.

Events moved slowly following the publication of *The Interpretation of Dreams*. The book received a number of reviews in specialized medical journals. Some were quite favorable, such as the comment in one journal that the book encompassed "many details of highly stimulating value, fine observations and theoretical outlook, and above all, extraordinarily rich material of very accurately recorded dreams." Others were skeptical. A few reviews expressing mixed opinions also appeared in the popular press. The book itself did not sell well—Freud was not well known, and *The Interpretation of Dreams* was difficult reading. The

Viennese medical community reacted to Freud's writing of this period
(Studies on Hysteria and *The Interpretation of Dreams)* either with
puzzled forbearance or the judgment that Freud's views were not to be
taken seriously. It certainly was not shocked by Freud's dwelling on
sexual matters. The publication in 1886 by Austrian psychiatrist Richard von Krafft-Ebing of his *Psychopathia Sexualis,* based on many case
histories of sexually abnormal individuals, had thoroughly inured the
medical world to perverse sexuality. Indeed Krafft-Ebing's work soon
reached a wider audience, and many novels and popular books on the
subject of sex were published in Austria and Germany around 1900.
Although Krafft-Ebing believed that Freud's theory of infant sexuality
(as presented in *Studies on Hysteria)* "sounded like a scientific fairy
tale," it did not prevent him from sponsoring Freud for the position of
professor extraordinarius at the University of Vienna, an appointment
that was granted in 1902. In all, the medical community tolerated
Freud.

Public reaction was somewhat more severe—in conventional Viennese society Freud's books were considered obscene, and his wife
Martha was pitied for having as a husband a man with such revolting
ideas. Stronger opposition from all strata of society, including the scientific, would come later.

During this period, Freud spent his time psychoanalyzing his eight
patients a day and writing. He would soon publish three new works,
The Psychopathology of Everyday Life on the unconscious basis of slips
of the tongue (Freudian slips) and memory lapses, *Wit and Its Relation
to the Unconscious,* and *Three Essays on the Theory of Sexuality* in
which he expanded his theory of infantile sexuality. By dint of his
appointment at the university, Freud was free to lecture there as he
chose. He used this opportunity to explain his views in his usual persuasive fashion to the general audience that came to hear him. Freud was
convinced by the unconscious material he was constantly seeing and
analyzing in his patients that he had discovered one of the great secrets
of nature, and he was unswervingly set on continuing his exploration of
the unconscious and advancing his ideas. In a letter to Fliess at the
time he described himself as a conquistador—with all the "inquisitive-
ness, daring and tenacity of such a man."

Freud's patients came from all over Europe. He was the physician of last resort in cases that others did not know how to approach. Freud's name slowly became known locally, and he attracted both physicians and nonmedical men who wanted to learn his methods. Alfred Adler and Wilhelm Stekel were two general practitioners in Vienna who came to Freud after reading *The Interpretation of Dreams.* In 1902, Stekel suggested to Freud that a discussion group be started. Freud liked the idea and shortly thereafter invited two doctors who were attending Freud's lectures to join Stekel, Adler, and himself in a Wednesday night discussion group at his home. This group was formalized as the Vienna Psychoanalytic Society in 1906. By 1911 it had become the Vienna chapter of the International Psychoanalytic Association.

The Wednesday night society expanded to about twenty members. Some were interested observers (one was a journalist, another a modern artist), but most were there to make the cause their own. Max Graf, a musicologist who attended, described the atmosphere as like that of the foundation of a religion. Freud was the prophet, and his pupils, inspired and convinced, were his apostles. Freud organized his group for the battle that was yet to be fought against society's opposition. There was to be no deviation from his teachings that might weaken his position. Graf observed: "Good hearted and considerate as he was in private life, Freud was hard and relentless in the presentation of his ideas. When the question of science came up he would break with his most intimate and reliable friends."

The Vienna Psychoanalytic Society was still active in 1921 when Abram Kardiner, a young American psychiatrist then being analyzed by Freud (and later a cofounder of the Columbia University School of Psychoanalysis), attended its meetings and described much the same atmosphere as in the earlier days.

The meetings of the Vienna Psychoanalytic Society were the most entertaining, especially that part of the evening devoted to discussion. This is where Freud showed his great mastery over people, and his great mastery over his subject matter.

Kardiner described one incident in particular in which a member of the society had just published a book on hypnosis. There was a great deal of criticism and heated discussion about what Freud had written on the subject:

> In the meanwhile, there was an enormous amount of discussion going on . . . about what Freud had said here, and what Freud had said there. . . . After the discussion had gone on for about an hour and a half, Freud tapped for order. He said words to the following effect:
> Gentlemen, you treat me with great dishonor. Why do you treat me as if I were already dead? Here you are, sitting among your-selves, discussing what I have said in this paper, what I have said in that paper, and there are quotations to and fro, and I am sitting at the head of the table and nobody so much as asks me "What did you really mean?" He said, "I take this to be an insult, and it worries me, because if this is what you do while I am still among you, I can well imagine what will happen when I am really dead."
> After this reproach, Freud abruptly adjourned the meeting.

The Vienna Society was Freud's own domain, and he had no serious intellectual opposition in the group. As we shall see, when an opposing view did arise, it inevitably resulted in the resignation of the man holding that view.

Between 1902 and 1908, Freud's works came to be read international-ally, and a small group of foreign psychiatrists were persuaded by his concepts. They were Ernest Jones in England, Abraham Brill in the United States, Karl Abraham in Germany, Sandor Ferenczi in Hun-gary, and Carl Jung in Switzerland. We will single out Jung for the moment.

When *The Interpretation of Dreams* first appeared in 1900, Jung was a twenty-five-year-old psychiatrist at the Burghölzli Psychiatric Hospital in Zurich. He was Swiss and came from a religious background (Jung's father was a small-town pastor). Jung had studied medicine at Basel University from 1895 to 1900, and then had gone directly to the Burghölzli Hospital as a resident. The Burghölzli was a large institution caring for some 3,000 mental patients of all varieties. Eugen Bleuler, its director, was an exceptionally skilled psychiatrist, devoted to his patients, and highly respected in medical circles. (Later in his career, Bleuler introduced the term "schizophrenia" and wrote *Dementia Praecox or the Group of Schizophrenias*—the definitive description of the disease.) Early in his residency, Jung read *The Interpretation of Dreams* and *Studies on Hysteria* and was intrigued by Freud's discoveries. He found his own evidence for repression and unconscious mental processes in tests he was performing at the Burghölzli on schizophrenic and hysteric patients. At Bleuler's suggestion, Jung had begun to use the Word Association Test, developed by the German psychologist Wilhelm Wundt. A patient was presented with a word and asked to reply with the first word that entered his or her mind. Jung found, as others had before, that the time of the patients' response was variable —it was longer when the patient's association to the presented word was unpleasant. Jung found in his patients that the words with longer reaction times were associated in a constellation or complex of memories that the patient had repressed. In hysterics, the complex was related to an old secret wound and could be abolished if the patient could be brought to face it—a finding similar to Freud's. In schizophrenics the complexes were irreversible.

Jung and other residents, with Bleuler's approval, started to use psychoanalysis at the Burghölzli. The Burghölzli was a progressive institution. Faced with the challenge and responsibility of treating thousands of mentally ill patients, Bleuler and Jung were eager to evaluate Freud's theory, which offered some rationale for mental illness and a method that might alleviate it. Besides the treatment of individual patients by individual physicians, there were staff conferences and discussions. In 1906 Jung sent Freud a copy of his newly published book on his word association studies. Jung also took the opportunity during that year to defend Freud's theory of hysteria at a psychiatric congress. In this defense, it was a portent of things to come that Jung expressed a view similar to that taken by Josef Breuer, namely that there was indeed a sexual basis for hysteria and that it was generally underestimated, but that this was not the only possible cause.

Jung met Freud for the first time early in 1907. He later related that

they talked for thirteen hours at their first meeting. The outcome of
the meeting was an alliance between the two men. Jung would join the
cause and be Freud's heir apparent. From Freud's viewpoint, Jung's
joining his ranks was a most welcome development. With his roots in
the mainstream of science and medicine, Freud did not enjoy his lonely
position outside the medical establishment. He felt, however, that he
had no choice—he had to follow the path in which his discoveries led.
And here was that very establishment in the form of Jung, Bleuler, and
the Burghölzli recognizing his work. Jung, on his part, felt that Freud
was a great man who had made a great discovery.

There was another reason for Freud's enthusiasm. Psychoanalysis was
a Jewish movement—Freud was a Jew as were most of his Viennese
followers. Freud was afraid that the cause in which he believed so
strongly, and which was coming under increasing attack for its content,
might be unfairly overwhelmed by anti-Semitism. (Freud expressed this
view in a letter to his German disciple Karl Abraham.) He saw in an
alliance with Jung the opportunity to overcome this handicap and have
psychoanalysis judged on its own merits. Freud was twenty years older
than Jung when they met—he was forty-nine and Jung was twenty-
nine—and under the circumstances Freud saw Jung as his natural suc-
cessor. Differences between the two men on the importance of infantile sexuality and other matters were apparent, but each for his own
reasons chose to minimize them. During the meeting Jung suggested
that a congress be convened the following year for all those interested
in psychoanalysis. Freud agreed, and Jung proceeded to organize the
first meeting of an international congress for psychoanalysts to be held
in Salzburg, Austria, in 1908. The meeting was duly held, Freud
presenting the main paper, and led to the founding of an international
organization. One outcome of the meeting was the decision to publish
a yearbook with Jung as editor and Freud and Bleuler as directors.

As an indication of his growing prominence, Freud was invited in
1909 to travel to the United States and provide a personal introduction
to his theories. The occasion was the twentieth anniversary of the
founding of Clark University in Worcester, Massachusetts. G. Stanley
Hall, a leading American psychologist and president of the university,
asked Freud to give a series of lectures as part of the celebration. Freud

traveled to America accompanied by Jung and Sandor Ferenczi, his Hungarian colleague, and was a guest in Hall's home during his stay. Besides the European psychoanalysts, American analyst Abraham Brill and Ernest Jones, who had settled in Toronto, were also in attendance. Leading members of American psychiatry, psychology, and other academic fields were present, including psychiatrist Adolf Meyer, psychologist William James, and anthropologist Franz Boas. Freud gave five lectures—his Five Lectures on Psychoanalysis—in which he described this early association with Breuer and how he was led by his observations to his theory of the unconscious and infantile sexuality. He was given an honorary degree, as was Jung. In his biography of Freud, Jones reports that Freud was visibly moved when he uttered the first words of his acceptance speech: "This is the first official recognition of our endeavors."

I pause here, coincident with Freud's explanations of his theories to his American audience, to bring the reader up to date on his developing ideas and summarize later additions he made to his theoretical framework. Freud wrote prolifically almost until the time of his death in 1939 (his collected works fill 23 volumes). I will consider only certain of his writings, those which contribute to my later discussion or provide the reader with pertinent background.

In *Three Essays on Sexuality,* published in 1905, and later works, Freud expanded his theory of infantile sexuality. He related certain additional observations and embedded them in libido theory, a concept he had introduced in earlier works. The concept of libido, based on an analogy with the physics of his day, involved the existence and flow of a quantity of psychic energy, which might be invested in or energize one mental activity or another. The preferred activity is sexual but the energy may be directed elsewhere.* In psychoanalytic writings, libido has also been conceptualized as a fluid that can be dammed up, discharged, or transferred from one psychic outlet to another. In the opinion of a number of psychoanalysts, libido theory is vague and has not proved to be productive. Others have found the concept to be of value in their view of psychological function. For our present purpose, in considering whether libido should be taken as a psychological finding to be explained on the basis of brain function, I believe it should not.

Its properties do not appear to be clearly established, and there is no indication that libido has a physiological counterpart in the brain.

I have raised the subject of libido at this point to give the reader an idea of the status of this central Freudian concept, since I will not be treating it later in my hypothesis. With this said, let us return to Freud's theory of infantile sexuality.

Freud elaborated on his theory of infant sexuality in the following way: The infant derives pleasure from the excitation of certain parts of the body—erogenous zones. Besides the genitals, these are the mouth, anus, and other skin surfaces. The child's sensual pleasure (sexual in Freud's view) is centered on each of these zones in sequence—oral, anal, and genital—as the child matures. The genital phase with the consequent normal adult sexuality will not be achieved if for some reason there is fixation at an earlier phase. Even with the genital phase achieved, there may be a predisposition in a given individual to regress to an earlier phase under certain circumstances. Further, although adult sexuality may not be overtly disturbed, there may be clusters of character traits in the adult that are derived from an oral or anal stage of development. Thus Freud described the anal-erotic character as being orderly, parsimonious, and obstinate. He explained that on the basis of his psychoanalytic observations, this was often related to an infantile predisposition to hold back stool and then obtain subsidiary pleasure from defecation.

Freud went on to say that psychic events were regulated in accordance with the "pleasure principle." In his view any given psychological process originated in an unpleasant state of tension. The psyche then sought a path that would reduce the tension to an optimal level.

In 1920, in an essay entitled "Beyond the Pleasure Principle," Freud changed his theory substantially. The First World War brought with it the traumatic neuroses of men exposed to trench warfare. These men had repeated dreams, reliving their traumatic experiences, and these dreams could no longer be contained within Freud's wish fulfillment theory. Freud introduced the concept of "compulsion to repetition," which he found more fundamental than the pleasure principle. This compulsion explained the traumatic dreams as well as hysterical attacks in which unpleasant events were repeated. (The dream was seen as "endeavoring to master the stimulus [traumatic event] retrospectively by developing the anxiety whose omission was the cause of the traumatic neurosis, that is to master the event by being active in the dream during the experience rather than experiencing it passively in an unprepared state as occurred originally.")

By this time Freud had identified the important process of transference, whereby the patient under psychoanalysis forms an intense emotional attachment to the analyst, which may take the form of love or hate, or may alternate. The analyst becomes a major participant in the patient's dreams, and the patient in the analysis tends to relive his early parental relationships with the analyst as a parent substitute. Freud saw this as another manifestation of the "compulsion to repetition."

In the framework of instinct theory, libido with its pleasure-seeking goals was now inadequate to explain this repetition of painful events such as traumatic dreams, so Freud introduced, to fill the gap, a new concept, the death instinct. Between libidinal instincts (now called Eros) and the death instinct, the latter was the more fundamental. There was "a tendency innate in living organic matter impelling it toward the reinstatement of an earlier condition," "the goal of life is death." From the death instinct Freud derived a primary aggressive drive. (He had previously explained aggression as an aspect of libido.) The postulate of the death instinct, seemingly based on nothing but the need to accommodate his theoretical framework to new observations, aroused opposition even among Freud's more devoted followers.

Freud's last major revision of theory was presented in 1923 in the work *The Ego and the Id*. Freud no longer found the classification of mental activity into conscious, preconscious, and unconscious categories sufficient. He introduced three new psychical entities, "Ego," "Superego," and "Id." The term "ego" was an old philosophical one denoting the entity through which the individual becomes aware of his own existence and the existence of the external world. If Freud had identified the ego with his conscious (and perhaps preconscious) domain, the superego (representing conscience) again with the conscious domain, and the id with the unconscious, the new classification would have been an uneventful elaboration. However, this would not have been consistent with other parts of his theory. To maintain the wish fulfillment theory of dreams, Freud had explained in *The Interpretation of Dreams* that punishment dreams were unconscious masochistic wishes, and now, in this new work, they became wishes of the conscience or superego. These wishes of the superego were unconscious, since it was not consciously known to the dreamer why the dream had its punishing quality. Thus while part of the superego was conscious (known feelings of guilt), another part was unconscious. Similarly Freud placed a large segment of the ego in the unconscious. Thus the unconscious censor in charge of repression was part of the ego—repression was a mechanism the ego used to defend itself against the impulses of the id. The id was, finally, the bedrock of the unconscious, a caldron of seething excitement, untamed passions, and destructive instincts.

Freud saw the id as the energizer of the entire psyche—the great "reservoir of the libido." As the infant developed, the ego grew out of the id. Thus:

The ego after all is only a portion of id, a portion that has been expediently modified by the proximity of the external world with its threat of danger. From a dynamic point of view it is weak, it has borrowed its energies from the id. . . . The ego must on the whole carry out the id's intentions, it fulfils its task by finding out the circumstances in which those intentions can best be achieved. The ego's relation to the id might be compared with that of a rider to his horse. The horse supplies the locomotive energy, while the rider has the privilege of deciding on the goal and of guiding the powerful animal's movement. But only too often there arises between the ego and the id the not precisely ideal situation of the rider being obliged to guide the horse along the path by which it itself wants to go.

We are warned by a proverb against serving two masters at the same time. The poor ego has things even worse: it serves three severe masters and does what it can to bring their claims and demands into harmony with one another. . . . Its three tyrannical masters are the external world, the super-ego and the id. When we follow the ego's efforts to satisfy them simultaneously—or rather, to obey them simultaneously—we cannot feel any regret at having personified this ego and having set it up as a separate organism. It feels hemmed in on three sides, threatened by three kinds of danger, to which, if it is hard pressed, it reacts by generating anxiety.

As we shall see, the plight of the ego and its defenses (the subject matter of ego psychology) is the predominant concern of psychoanalysis today.

However metaphorically appealing some of Freud's concepts may have been (and may be), there were clear excesses of theory—such as, in the opinion of most psychoanalysts, the death instinct. The net result was a mixture of observations and layers of hypotheses from which it will be our task to select those parts which may fairly be taken as our psychological data.

To return to our history of psychoanalysis, following his American trip, Freud proceeded to the next step, organizing his movement. The International Psychoanalytic Association was formed at a congress held in Nuremberg in 1910, and on Freud's initiative, over the objections of the Vienna circle, Jung was elected president. A few months after the formation of the association, the first of a series of defections from Freud's ranks began. Eugen Bleuler, head of the Burghölzli, though continuing to believe in Freud's discoveries, resigned because of what he regarded as Freud's unscientific attitude in not allowing dissenting opinions to be heard within the association. Bleuler's views were beautifully expressed in a letter to Freud:

Scientifically I still do not understand why for you it is so important that the whole edifice [of psychoanalysis] should be accepted. But I remember I told you once that no matter how great your scientific accomplishments are, psychologically you impress me as an artist. From this point of view it is understandable that you do not want your art product to be destroyed. In art we have a unit which cannot be torn apart. In science you made a great discovery which has to stay. How much of what is loosely connected with it will survive is not important.

Within a year, Freud forced the resignation of Alfred Adler, a founding member of the Vienna Society, and five others who sympathized with the new ideas Adler was advocating. These ideas constituted the first reformulation of Freud's theories.

Adler did not use Freud's method of having a patient lie on a couch, the analyst behind him, and free associate. Adler sat in a chair facing his patient. Although one might imagine that the amount of free association might be limited in this situation, by delving into memories and dreams, Adler obtained from his patients unconscious material similar to that seen by Freud. Adler's interpretations were quite different however. As Adler saw it, the child viewed life as a struggle, first for security and then for power, and evolved a strategy to that end. The Oedipal complex was not universal in the young boy. When it did occur, it resulted from excessive pampering by the mother, and it did not constitute primarily a sexual attraction to the mother but rather a power struggle in which the boy tried to surpass his father. (Should the father be pampering, the child would turn predominantly toward him.) The spoiled child was sexually precocious because he learned to deny himself nothing. The sexual pleasure the young boy did associate with his mother was secondary to his satisfaction in dominating her. Adler believed that Freud had taken the pampered child, worked out the unconscious dynamics of its strivings for sexual gratification, and then considered these dynamics universal. But the striving for sexual gratification was only one of the countless varieties of strivings and was not the central motivation of all personalities.

Adler originated the term "inferiority complex." In the struggle for survival and power, the child may have developed deep-seated feelings of inadequacy and inferiority. These may have arisen from an "organ inferiority," an actual physical weakness or deformity in childhood, or such feelings may have been induced by a lack of parental tenderness or parental ridicule of a child's feelings. (The origin of Adler's idea of "organ inferiority" was apparent. He had rickets as a child of two, and was sickly for a period thereafter.) A reaction to these feelings of inferiority could be an exalted and unrealistic fantasy of superiority.

Adler believed that the nuclear form of an individual's adaptation to life, the "prototype," was set down by the age of four and was difficult to change thereafter. The goal of Adler's "individual therapy" was nonetheless to aid in this adaptation to life—to analyze feelings of inferiority and to instill courage. He analyzed childhood memories to this end. He believed dreams reflected ongoing waking life; they revealed the adaptational "life situation" goals and problems of the individual. Adler encountered resistance and transference in all of his patients as did Freud, but considered these impediments to treatment, to be pointed out as undesirable and eradicated. Adler stressed another aspect of adaptation, the ability of the individual to relate to the community. We shall see that Adler's ideas reappeared in the theories of neo-Freudian psychoanalysts in the 1930s and 1940s and that Freudian psychoanalysts came to deal with the same material via ego psychology.

Although Adler's work may have contributed new interpretive insights into the human personality, for our present purpose of establishing a body of psychological observations that we may say are valid, his work neither adds nor subtracts very much from what we have noted thus far. Unconscious memories, the Oedipal complex, resistance (repression), and transference were all present.

The next defection was a source of deep disappointment to Freud—the defector was Jung, and the reason again was a difference in interpretation, which developed into personal animosity. Jung, now president of the International Psychoanalytic Association, was formulating his own theories and turning against infantile sexuality. As an example, Jung reduced the role of the Oedipal complex from the sexual to the demand for love from the father and the mother. Jung returned from a second trip to the United States where he presented his views. On November 14, 1912, Freud wrote:

Dear Dr. Jung *[all previous correspondence had carried the salutation "Dear Friend"]*,

I greet you on your return from America, no longer as affectionately as on the last occasion in Nuremburg—you have successfully broken me of that habit—but still with considerable sympathy, interest, and satisfaction at your personal success. Many thanks for your news of the state of affairs in America. But we know that the battle will not be decided over there. You have reduced a good

deal of resistance with your modifications, but I shouldn't advise
you to enter this in the credit column because, as you know, the
farther you remove yourself from what is new in ψA [psychoanaly-
sis], the more certain you will be of applause and the less resistance you will meet.

Jung's reply was:

15 November 1912

Dear Professor Freud *[his customary greeting]*,
    Your letter, just arrived, has evoked in me a ψA attitude which
seems to be the only right one at the moment. I shall continue to
go my own way undaunted.

A meeting attempting a reconciliation and a series of letters followed, in which Jung grew ever more restive at what he saw as Freud's
underestimation of his accomplishments and efforts at control. By December, Jung had grown virulent in his attack on Freud. Thus:

1003 Seestrasse, Kusnach-Zurich,
18 December 1912

Dear Professor Freud,
    May I say a few words to you in earnest? I admit the ambiva-
lence of my feelings towards you, but am inclined to take an
honest and absolutely straightforward view of the situation. If you
doubt my word, so much the worse for you. I would, however,
point out that your technique of treating your pupils like patients
is a blunder. In that way you produce either slavish sons or impu-
dent puppies (Adler-Stekel and the whole insolent gang now
throwing their weight about in Vienna). I am objective enough to
see through your little trick. You go around sniffing out all the
symptomatic actions in your vicinity, thus reducing everyone to
the level of sons and daughters who blushingly admit the existence
of their faults. Meanwhile you remain on top as the father, sitting
pretty. For sheer obsequiousness nobody dares to pluck the

prophet by the beard and inquire for once what you would say to a patient with a tendency to analyse the analyst instead of himself. You would certainly ask him: "Who's got the neurosis?" . . . You know, of course, how far a patient gets with self-analysis: not out of his neurosis—just like you. If ever you should rid yourself entirely of your complexes and stop playing the father to your sons and instead of aiming continually at their weak spots took a good look at your own for a change, then I will mend my ways and at one stroke uproot the vice of being in two minds about you. . . .

I shall continue to stand by you publicly while maintaining my own views, but privately shall start telling you in my letters what I really think of you. I consider this procedure only decent.

No doubt you will be outraged by this peculiar token of friendship, but it may do you good all the same.

With best regards,

Most sincerely yours, Jung

Freud's reply was the last letter he wrote to Jung:

Vienna, 3 January 1913

Dear Mr. President,
Dear Doctor,

. . . I can answer only one point in your previous letter in any detail. Your allegation that I treat my followers like patients is demonstrably untrue. In Vienna, I am reproached for the exact opposite. . . .

Otherwise your letter cannot be answered. It creates a situation that would be difficult to deal with in a personal talk and totally impossible in correspondence. It is a convention among us analysts that none of us need feel ashamed of his own bit of neurosis. But one who while behaving abnormally keeps shouting that he is normal gives ground for the suspicion that he lacks insight into his illness. Accordingly, I propose that we abandon our personal relations entirely. I shall lose nothing by it, for my only emotional tie with you has long been a thin thread—the lingering effect of past disappointments—and you have everything to gain, in view of the remark you recently made in Munich, to the effect that an intimate relationship with a man inhibited your scientific freedom. I therefore say, take your full freedom and spare me your supposed "tokens of friendship." We are agreed that a man should subordinate his personal feelings to the general interests of his branch of endeavour. You will never have reason to complain of any lack of correctness on my part where our common undertaking and the pursuit of scientific aims are concerned; I may say, no more reason in the future than in the past. On the other hand, I am entitled to expect the same from you.

Regards,

Yours sincerely, Freud

After a series of political maneuvers, in April 1914 Jung resigned from the International Association, took the Zurich members with him, and founded a new school of analytical psychology.

Jung's revision of Freud's theory was on several levels. Closest to direct unconscious material and its interpretation was his view of infant sexuality. Jung did not deny the role of sexuality but classified it as just one of the infant's instinctual drives. Thus, in a lecture at Fordham University in New York City in 1912, Jung denied the essential element of Freud's theory that all infantile gratification was sexual:

Freud points to the unmistakable excitement and satisfaction of the infant while sucking, and he compares the emotional mechanisms with those of the sexual act. This comparison leads him to assume that the act of sucking has a sexual quality. . . . [But] if Freud derives the sexual quality of the act of sucking from the analogy of the emotional mechanism, biological experience would also justify a terminology qualifying the sexual act as a function of nutrition. This is exceeding the bound in both directions.

Jung hastened to point out that Freud did not consider sucking exclusively a manifestation of the sexual instinct but a sort of combination of nutritional and sexual instincts, and that the side-by-side existence of hunger and sex obviously exists in the adult. He continued:

> We deceive ourselves if we think that the two instincts exist side by side in the infant, for then we project into the psyche of the child an observation taken over from the psychology of adults. The co-existence or separate manifestation of the two instincts is not found in the infant, for one of the instinctual systems is not developed at all or is quite rudimentary. If we take the attitude that [any] striving for pleasure is something sexual, we might just as well say, paradoxically, that hunger is a sexual striving, since it seeks out pleasure by satisfaction. But if we juggle concepts like that, we should have to allow our opponents to apply the terminology of hunger to sexuality.

Then in a comment obviously condescending to Freud:

> This kind of one-sidedness appears over and over again in the history of science. I am not saying this as a reproach: on the contrary, we must be glad that there are people who are courageous enough to be immoderate and one-sided. It is to them that we owe our discoveries. What is regrettable is that each should defend his one-sidedness so passionately. Scientific theories themselves are merely suggestions as to how things might be observed.

As already noted, Jung minimized the Oedipus complex, especially its sexual content. Thus:

> The term Oedipus complex naturally does not mean conceiving this conflict in its adult form [as in the Greek myth], but rather on a reduced scale suitable for childhood. All it means, in effect, is that the childish demands for love are directed to mother and father, and to the extent that these demands have already attained a certain degree of intensity, so that the chosen object is jealously defended, we can speak of an Oedipus complex.

Jung believed that there were patients whose psychological organization was indeed derived from cravings for instinctual gratification and
others whose psychological structure was best described by Adler's will
to power. Indeed he implied that Freud and Adler had each come upon
his theory because it described each man's own psyche. (Freud, the
adored first son of a beautiful, young mother, developed strong Oedipal
feelings and was sensitive to these in his patients; Adler, having suffered from rickets as a child, was sensitive to questions of inferiority
and power.) Jung differed markedly from Freud in his view of neurosis.
As we have seen, Freud carefully worked out the unresolved Oedipal
conflicts leading to neurosis. His view was that the Oedipal conflict was
universal, but recognized that it resulted in neurosis only in some individuals. Freud ascribed this tendency to neurosis (especially in hysteria)
to an inherent predisposition. Jung, confronting the same question in
his own practice, saw neurosis as almost completely an innate psychological deficiency. Thus:

> The ultimate and deepest root of neurosis appears to be the innate
> sensitiveness, which causes difficulties even to the infant at the
> mother's breast, in the form of unnecessary excitement and resis-
> tance.

Jung believed neurotics possessed an innate oversensitivity, which
induced a flight from reality and a regression into fantasy. The result
was that in the neurotic, unconscious material which was present in
everyone (and would ordinarily underlie the development of certain
personality characteristics) came to dominate the entire psyche.

At this point, Jung's ideas departed from psychology and medicine
and entered the realm of philosophy and religion. Besides psychological
forces, Jung postulated something deeper in the psyche—the spirit. He
states:

> I do not doubt that the natural instincts or drives are forces of
> propulsion in psychic life, whether we call them sexuality or will to
> power; but neither do I doubt that these instincts come into colli-
> sion with the spirit, for they are continually colliding with some-

thing, and why should not this something be called spirit. My attitude toward all religions is therefore a positive one.

In his final formulation, Jung proposed a theory of the mind that entered the mystical. According to Jung, a collective psyche, handed down from earliest man, constituted the deepest stratum of each individual's mind. Within the collective psyche and thus within each person's mind, were archetypes of God, a feminine figure (which was in the minds of men as well as women, giving rise to the feminine part of man's nature), a masculine figure, (the wise old man), and the mother. The universal quality of myths in different cultures was explained as resulting from the same archetypes being present in the minds of all men throughout history. Jung went so far as to state that certain basic ideas of physics such as the conservation of energy were archetypal with only certain conditions needed for them to appear. According to Jung, these conditions were present for Robert Mayer, a physician, in 1884 when he enunciated the theory of the conservation of energy for the first time. How did the collective psyche originate and by what means was it transmitted from one generation to the next? Jung did not say how it originated, but thought that Lamarckian inheritance of ideas might be responsible for its transmission.

Jung's stated method of therapy revolved around his theory. A patient in Jungian analysis, as in Adlerian, sat facing the analyst. Dreams were used extensively but free association was not—rather the patient was asked to put him or herself in the dream situation and then expand on possible meanings of the dream images. Various stages of the analysis proceeded as the individual's own concerns were expressed in his dreams. In the final stage this presumably led to the unearthing of the patient's archetypal figures. Contrary to this theoretical scenario for unraveling a patient's psyche, Jung, who was an unusually skilled therapist, was known not to adhere to this method but treated each patient differently. His general approach was to make the patient aware of his current situation and to have the patient apply the therapeutic insights thus gained to his practical life. As might be expected, Jung also encouraged a sense of spiritual value.

Jung's work does not change our list of psychological phenomena as observed by Freud in any major regard. Jung found in his patients unconscious mental processes and repression as did Freud, and he certainly agreed with Freud as to the importance of symbols in dreams. Jung also stated that he encountered transference in every patient he treated. Jung's interpretations were of course different from Freud's. He believed transference was a destructive phenomenon, degrading to the patient and potentially dangerous to the psychotherapist because of the overvaluation the patient placed on his therapist (Jung was the first to emphasize that an analyst had to undergo his own analysis before treating patients). Jung also believed that dreams represented considerably more than wish fulfillments, and we will have occasion to return to Jung's theory of dreams in the last section of this book. Finally, Jung's criticism of Freud's theory of infant sexuality was cogent and his change of emphasis on the etiology of neurosis a serious recasting of Freud's view.

Where did Jung get his fanciful ideas of archetypal figures and the collective unconscious, concepts that can hardly be taken seriously today? All indications are that they were derived from Jung's own psyche. His autobiography emphasizes Jung's early preoccupation with religious imagery and the appearance in his earliest dreams of images easily interpreted as archetypal. Thus one may say that Jung joined Freud and Adler in formulating his theory of the unconscious to encompass the material he found in his own psyche.

Jung resigned as president of the International Psychoanalytical Association in 1914, and Freud once again took control of the organization. That same year saw the outbreak of the First World War. At that time psychoanalysis was still a minor part of psychiatry in Europe and the United States, disparaged by most of the medical community. The war was a turning point for psychoanalysis. Under the conditions of trench warfare—days of bombardment waiting for an order to attack, followed by fierce combat—increasing numbers of men succumbed to war neuroses. There was a resurgence of hysterical paralyses, phobias, and obsessions. There were also the recurrent dreams of traumatic combat experiences. Neurologists and psychiatrists were assigned to military hospitals to treat these cases. They found that Freud's was the only theory applicable and psychoanalysis the only treatment promising a cure. Due to wartime conditions, only a small number of patients were psychoanalyzed, but in the large military hospitals, just as at the Burghölzli, Freud's ideas became the center of discussion. The net effect was to press home to medical people and laymen alike the importance of unconscious mental processes. Following the war, the status of psychoanalysis grew rapidly, especially in the United States. Abraham Brill and Ernest Jones (in Canada) had labored diligently to prepare the groundwork—Brill had founded the New York Psychoanalytic Association in 1911 and Jones the American Psychoanalytic Association (for analysts in other cities in the United States) during the same year. Soon after the war a new contingent of American psychiatrists were in Vienna being analyzed by Freud. One of them was Abram Kardiner whom I mentioned earlier. These analysts returned to the United States to start their own practices.

There was no other cure for neurosis, so patients turned to psychoanalysis. Discussion grew in medical circles and in the popular press, and by the late 1920s Freudian ideas were on the way toward dominating American psychiatry. In describing that period, Morton Prince (who had treated Miss Beauchamp for multiple personality) wrote:

Freudian psychology had flooded the field like a rising tide, and the rest of us were left submerged like clams buried in the sands at low tide.

At this point I interrupt our history of psychoanalysis to describe an aspect of it which we have not yet considered—the way it has actually been practiced.

An example of how psychoanalysis was carried out by Freud was provided by Kardiner, who in 1976 described his own analysis with Freud. The year was 1921. Freud was analyzing several young foreign candidates, among them Kardiner, grateful that his fees were being paid in hard currency in inflation-ridden Vienna. Kardiner did not suffer from any classical neurosis or other outstanding psychological impairment. He undertook his analysis for training purposes—yet he looked to it to reveal the unconscious basis for certain feelings and personality characteristics that he wanted to change.

Kardiner was thirty years old at the time of his analysis. He had grown up in a very poor family on the lower East Side of New York, had lost his mother at the age of three, acquired a beautiful and seductive stepmother at the age of three and a half, had gone through a youthful phase of shame at being a Jew, suffered debilitating anxiety at schoolwork for a while, had managed these problems, gone through college and medical school, and was now a psychiatrist. He had an active sexual interest in women (during the analysis he dreamed of having sexual intercourse with his stepmother), and his main complaint was a feeling that he carried with him since his childhood—a feeling of being a nobody and not having enough aggression to envy anyone else, even when such envy would be only natural.

Kardiner's analysis lasted six months, five sessions a week. Freud took an active part in interpreting Kardiner's dreams and free associations and, according to Kardiner, was brilliant at it. (At one point Freud managed to discover from a dream the cause of a phobia of masks that Kardiner had acquired in childhood. It related to Kardiner finding his mother dead at the age of three, a memory that he had repressed but later verified.) Freud talked in direct terms and did not use abstract theoretical formulations. All of the psychoanalytic material arose from dreams, memories, and events that Kardiner brought up. In the course of Kardiner's analysis, Freud's interpretations led to the Oedipus complex and to unconscious homosexuality. Kardiner accepted the interpretation of his Oedipus complex but not that of homosexuality, although a considerable part of the analysis was spent on this matter. Comparing notes with other psychiatrists in training, Kardiner discovered that the Oedipus complex and unconscious homosexuality was a routine part of everyone's analysis. What transpired in the psychoanalysis as a result of these revelations? Kardiner comments:

Once he located the Oedipus complex and worked through the unconscious homosexuality, there wasn't anything much left to do. One unscrambled the patient and let him scramble it together as best he could by himself. And if he didn't do it, Freud would give him a couple of barbs every now and then to encourage him and to hasten matters. Freud really did not know very much about

Durcharbeitung [working through], as we now understand it, though it subsequently became the essential task of the therapeutic process.

In retrospect, writing in 1976, Kardiner was dissatisfied with his analysis. He felt it left his personality unaltered in the one area most important to him. Thus:

Freud's perspective on the whole problem of development was constricted by his emphasis on unconscious homosexuality and the Oedipus Complex. He could have helped me develop self-assertion and, with a little encouragement, this could have been easy because I had a good deal of drive. By making it into a problem of unconscious homosexuality, he turned my attention to a non-existent problem and away from a very active one.

Kardiner's analysis raises all the basic issues of psychoanalysis—how much analysis of dreams, how much free association, who interprets the unconscious material, analyst or patient, and to what extent and finally, under what circumstances does insight lead to change?

Freud developed psychoanalysis as a treatment for neurosis, and as we shall see later in this chapter, even in his own hands cure was by no means always forthcoming. The patient population changed through the years. More and more persons such as Kardiner without classical neurosis were analyzed. At the same time neuroses themselves seemed to change. The incidence of hysteria dropped markedly—obsessional neuroses became more resistant to treatment. In Freud's view and experience, incomplete resolution of the Oedipus complex led to sexual conflicts and neuroses, and by uncovering these conflicts, psychoanalysis might effect a cure. As time went by, analysts came to see that Oedipal conflicts as well as other conflicts such as those associated with an infantile fear of abandonment (fear for security as sensed by Adler), though perhaps not resulting in outright neuroses, constituted the substrate of the entire personality. Psychoanalysis grew longer—it did not take six months but, as is typical today, six or more years. Beyond uncovering the unconscious material (which seemed to be ever more difficult) there came the major task of analysis, the "working through." This involved using the transference relationship in which the subject felt and lived out his conflicts, substituting the analyst for other important people in his early life. The object of the "working through" was to have the subject go beyond an understanding of his unconscious ideas and motivations, to a desired change in personality.

The form that Freudian psychoanalysis takes today, then, is an analysis of how the character develops, how the ego (as defined by Freud) accommodates to its "three harsh masters"—the id, the superego, and the real world. To describe this, a theory of ego psychology was developed by Freud's followers in the 1940s, notable among them being Anna Freud, Erik Erikson, and Heinz Hartmann.* Erik Erikson, in presenting his concept of ego psychology, inspected the manifest content of dreams anew and stated that the manifest content was not a "mere shell to the kernel—the latent dream" but that its style of representation showed all of the ego's defenses, compromises and achievements. In the case of Freud's Irma dream for example, beyond the wish to be held blameless for Irma's condition, Erikson saw an expression of Freud's conscience (guilt over not curing Irma in real life), anxieties as to his abilities, and his means of coping by appealing to higher authority (Breuer in the guise of Dr. M.).

Turning back to psychoanalytic history, events leading to the Second World War hastened the shift of the center of psychoanalysis from Middle Europe to England and especially to the United States. Freud himself left Vienna for England in 1938, a year before his death. Public awareness was brought to a high pitch in the United States not only by the assimilation of psychoanalytic concepts with their natural appeal to the imagination into the arts and media, but by the promulgation of new theories of the psyche by analysts such as Karen Horney, Eric Fromm, and Harry Stack Sullivan—the neo-Freudians. Their theories addressed themselves to the factors influencing personality development. These analysts continued to use Freudian terminology but their explanations were more closely related to those of Adler—the more important determinants of personality were the child's need for security and affection, the struggle for power and the effects of interrelationships among people, and society's influence on the individual. In their psychoanalytically oriented treatments, theory became almost irrelevant. Treatment depended on the skill of the therapist and on its structured form, that is, whether it was psychoanalysis, complete with lying on the couch, dream analysis, and free association, or a less rigid type of talking therapy.

From our present perspective of establishing a psychological framework for future use, the work of these later analysts tended to confirm that ego structure with many characteristics determined by unconscious forces was set down in early childhood. On the specific identification of phenomena such as transference, repression, and the Oedipus complex, nothing new was added. Neo-Freudians found transference and repression in their patients. The Oedipus complex was identified in some but was interpreted on a basis other than infantile sexuality.

By the 1950s psychoanalysis had become the major influence in American psychiatry. It was the only comprehensive theory of the psyche available and seemed to hold out great hope as a therapeutic tool. Since the 1960s though, a transformation has taken place, so that today psychoanalysis is a small, specific discipline within psychiatry with its own unique applications and goals. To understand this transformation I want to consider now the views of the critics of psychoanalysis.

These critics argue that psychoanalytic theory is unscientific and that its therapy is largely ineffective. They variously conclude that although unconscious mental processes may in fact affect man's motivations and actions, psychoanalysis has not come to grips with the matter—or that, though there may well be an unconscious, it is conscious thought and will alone that determine man's behavior.

In evaluating the scientific or unscientific nature of Freudian theory, we first note that Freud developed his theory in several stages. In light of the difficulty of precise definition in the entire field of psychology, certain of Freud's formulations in *The Interpretation of Dreams* were not unreasonable. It is generally accepted today that there is an unconscious—that is, there are memories and thoughts not available for conscious recall. Clearly, dreams are distorted compared to waking thought, and Freud hypothesized mechanisms (condensation, displacement, representability, symbolism) to account for the distortion. Repression is an understandable concept. (It was independently arrived at by Jung through use of word association tests.) Whether or not repression is operative in dream formation in keeping instinctual impulses from conscious awareness is an unresolved question, but the concept can be defined and is possibly open to future investigation. When it came to interpreting the meaning of dreams, however, Freud's theory grew more difficult to pin down. As we have seen, he proposed that dreams were wish fulfillments. If all dreams had fallen neatly into this category, this hypothesis might have been persuasive. However, when Freud sought to explain dreams that were clearly punishment or anxiety ridden as wish-fulfilling by bringing in such concepts as wishes of the superego and the death instinct, the cogency of his argument was lost. There was no way to define adequately or prove the existence of these other entities, and one had the impression that Freud was straining to maintain a unifying, simple explanation as he had done previously when he had insisted that infantile sexuality was, without exception, the basis of hysteria. Problems also arose in the interpretation of individual dreams. The Oedipal dream of killing the father and sexually possessing the mother was interpreted by Freud as a sexual drama and by Adler as a struggle for power, and there was no conceivable way to determine which of the interpretations was correct.

As Freud continued to add one idea on top of another, psychoanalytic theory became more and more obscure. Freud's theoretical ideas continued to expand, and soon psychoanalysis was rendered unscientific in the most basic sense—there was no conceivable manner in which it could be tested. That is, the theory became so broad that regardless of what psychological event might occur, psychoanalytic theory could find a way to explain it. As a result, the theory could not be refuted by any psychological observation and hence was untestable. For example, in 1926 the concept of "reaction formation" was introduced by Freud to describe a defense mechanism of the ego by which the ego might react in one of two opposite ways to an unconscious impulse arising in the id. The unconscious feelings of envy and jealousy in a daughter toward her mother might result in hostile behavior. On the other hand, an unconscious reaction formation of the ego against these feelings might set in, and the daughter would then act with exaggerated tenderness and concern toward her mother. An analyst finding such unconscious hostility in dream material (the Electra complex, a female counterpart of the Oedipus complex) and observing hostile behavior toward the mother in real life might conclude that the unconscious thoughts resulted in the behavior. (In terms of a test, the analyst would predict that the hostile behavior results from the unconscious material, and psychoanalytic theory would be confirmed.) On the other hand, if he observed tenderness and kindly behavior, he might say that a reaction formation had taken over—once again the theory would be confirmed. However, the argument might well be put forth with no independent means of verifying the reaction formation—it would be an assumption introduced to explain a contrary result.* The assumption might represent the true state of affairs but there would be no way to prove it. As Ernest Nagel, philosopher of science, put it:

> One is therefore led to imagine . . . whether there are any statements which are unmistakable instances of deductions from Freudian theory or whether the theory has the remarkable feature that a statement can be shown to be a theorem only if it is first accepted as a postulate . . . there is good ground for supposing that Freudian theory can always be so manipulated that it escapes refutation no matter what the well-established facts may be.

Philosopher Karl Popper expressed similar statements in discussing Freud's and Adler's theories:

> The two psychoanalytic theories . . . were simply nontestable, irrefutable. There was no conceivable human behavior which could contradict them. This does not mean that Freud and Adler were not seeing certain things correctly: I personally do not doubt that much of what they say is of considerable importance, and may well play its part one day in a psychological science which is testable. But it does mean that those clinical observations which analysts naively believe confirm their theory cannot do this any more than the daily confirmations which astrologers find in their practice. And so for Freud's epic of the Ego, the Super-ego and

the Id, no substantially stronger claim for scientific status can be made for it than Homer's collected stories from Olympus. They contain most interesting psychological suggestions, but not in any testable form.

Psychoanalysis is not a science, and there are few analysts today who would consider it so; as we shall see, its skillful practice may be considered an art. It has not, over time, progressed by the continuing testing of hypotheses as do the most advanced sciences. But, in defense of psychoanalysis, this is hardly to be considered a condemnation. It would be most surprising if psychoanalysis, dealing as it does with the complexity of human thought and behavior, had progressed to the state of the physical sciences where elements may be scrutinized and experimented upon in isolation. Rather, psychoanalysis is in an early stage, passed through by all sciences, in which observations are gathered and connections are sought to related bodies of knowledge. In psychoanalysis, the gathering of observations has its special characteristics. It consists of many bits of evidence, dreams, free associations, reactions during the transference relationship, all interrelated and converging to make the same psychological point, and so convince the analyst and patient of its validity. Indeed, in a given case, reaction formation may not be an unsubstantiated speculation. A patient may dream directly of hating her mother and in the dream decide to act meekly toward her out of fear. Or a loving daughter may express hatred for her mother in an uncontrolled outburst during an analytic session. The use of reaction formation, Oedipus complex, or other psychoanalytically derived concepts to explain an individual's behavior with incomplete evidence may be little more than a parlor game, but that is not to say that such unconscious constellations of thoughts and motivations have not been revealed by patients in psychoanalysis. The difficulty with these data of psychoanalysis is extracting them in verifiable form from the psychoanalytic sessions in which they occur, sessions where the goal is primarily therapeutic and not investigatory.

Despite these problems, as I have noted, certain psychoanalytic concepts have been widely reported and are sufficiently well defined to be included in our psychological data for later comparison with brain function. These are dream distortion, repression, and transference.

Psychoanalysts have not been unaware of these problems with analytic theory. Convinced by their clinical practice of the reality and potency of unconscious mental forces, some analysts have been bluntly critical of psychoanalytic theory and are attempting to put it on a firmer footing. Thus psychoanalyst Emanuel Peterfreund states:

> Psychoanalysis has innumerable basically valid clinical empirical generalizations. These represent the clinical facts of observation and the relationships among them . . . [but] because of its basically hydrodynamic character [libido theory], its primitive anthropomorphism [ego, id, superego], and its fundamental conceptual divorce from all of evolutionary time, current psychoanalytic theory is a very limited theory. It cannot develop an adequate learning theory or an adequate theory of the psychoanalytic process, and it cannot be meaningfully linked to modern neurophysiology.

Peterfreund's research is directed at developing an information-systems theory for the clinical data of psychoanalysis. (Information-systems theory, arising from computer science, deals with the logic of information handling and decision making.)

Several other lines of investigation have been carried out by psychoanalysts. In the area of the meaning of dreams, psychoanalysts have recognized the inadequacy of wish fulfillment as an explanation and have suggested other hypotheses based on their own psychoanalytic cases. These hypotheses largely center on the idea that dreams are involved in the adaptation to or the solution of focal problems in the current life of the dreamer. These analysts conclude that certain dreams are indeed wishful solutions to these problems; others are a search for a solution or an adaptive response based on the experience of the dreamer from childhood onward.*

Attempts have been made to test some of the general conclusions of Freudian theory such as the idea that male homosexuality results from unconscious fears arising from the Oedipus complex. A family constellation consisting of an overbearing and seductive mother and weak or

detached father would, according to the theory, be conducive to homosexuality. An extensive study of 106 male homosexuals and 100 male
heterosexuals (control subjects) undergoing psychoanalysis, published
in 1962, found that although this family constellation did constitute
the background of most of their homosexual subjects, there were men
in their heterosexual group with similar backgrounds. There were other
unknown determining factors for homosexuality.

Although one cannot draw a causal link between unconscious Oedipal conflicts and homosexuality, reports of analysts quite cognizant of
the pitfalls of their field (such as patient suggestibility and overinter-
pretation by the analyst) indicate that this material does appear. A
subject may be an "obligatory" homosexual, addicted to cruising and
picking up casual sexual partners, perhaps even while living with another homosexual partner. The subject may dream directly of having
his father's penis inserted into his anus (the subject and father at their
actual ages) and may, via free association, without any suggestion or
interpretation by the analyst, find that this means to him the gaining of
his father's sexual strength for his own. The need for this gratification
drives him to periodic homosexual acts.

Psychoanalysts have also used systematic observations to study
mother-infant and mother-child relationships and have defined a number of steps in the young child's psychological growth.* Lastly, and
most interesting from my point of view, is the recent expression in
psychoanalytic and psychiatric writings that the time may be appropriate to try to link psychoanalytic observations with brain function and
thus establish the basis for psychoanalysis as an experimental science.*
My hypothesis is, of course, an attempt in this direction.

Putting theory aside, it is psychoanalysis as a therapy that has determined its course from the 1950s to the present. Freud himself was not
optimistic about therapy. He pointed out that psychoanalysis was best
used for "small neuroses" and reported few therapeutically successful
cases in his own writings. Most of the patients he used as illustrative
examples admittedly were not cured. Nevertheless, in the enthusiasm
of the 1950s, and with no other therapy available, psychoanalysis was
used to treat a wide variety of psychiatric illnesses such as schizophrenia, manic-depressive psychosis, and depression, with virtually no suc-

cess. Experience was similar in attempts to treat such psychologically associated disorders as drug and alcohol addiction. Major neuroses such as well-developed obsessional neuroses and more recently narcissistic character disorders were also found to be resistant to treatment.

At the same time new methods of treatment became available. Foremost among them was the use of psychoactive drugs which will be discussed in some detail later in this book. Other forms of talking therapy were developed that were shorter and less expensive than psychoanalysis, in addition to techniques such as behavior modification, which was somewhat effective in minor neuroses such as phobias. In view of the therapeutic failings of psychoanalysis, psychiatrists and other mental health professionals turned to these methods to help their patients.

As the situation stabilized during the years following the rash of wide-ranging attempts at treating many mental disorders, psychoanalysis settled into the position it presently occupies. To close this chapter, I will describe the state of psychoanalysis today.

About 2,000 psychiatrists belong to the American Psychoanalytic Association (membership in the American Psychiatric Association is 32,000), and there are at least a like number of psychologists who practice psychoanalysis in its original form today. A major segment of the patient population is made up of psychiatrists and other mental health professionals who see it as a means of continued education and training. A survey in 1972 of 140 East Coast analysts elicited the response that over half of their patients were in the mental health field. The same survey showed that 32 percent of the subjects were independently wealthy (a six-year analysis may cost upward of $70,000 and many analyses extend to ten and twelve years). A certain number of subjects are accepted at low fees and are analyzed by analysts-in-training under supervision. The majority of subjects possess, like Abram Kardiner, what might be termed the normal range of psychological problems.

Psychoanalysis is also applied in some other areas. It may be the treatment of choice for problems of character disorder if the patient has a sufficiently strong ego. Neuroses are also treated, but many long-term neurotics are considered poor psychoanalytic risks. A small group of analysts specializes in homosexuality. The objective of the treatment here is either to help the subject understand and overcome his conflicts regarding his homosexuality or, in a lesser number of cases, to precipitate a change to heterosexuality.

What happens during psychoanalysis? Given that the patient lies on a couch, what then occurs is highly variable. How much free association, dream interpretation, how the transference is used—these are all in the hands of the analyst. Thus analytic practice is very much an art. The points are often subtle. Should one treat the patient with a certain degree of warmth (as did Freud) or maintain a complete barrier to communication other than through the rules of analysis—that is, no question as to the analyst's interests, opinions, or personal life is answered except perhaps to ask why the patient wants to know. A current debate centers on the appropriate response of the analyst when he hears, say, that the patient's father has died. One side considers the proper response to be a normal expression of sympathy—to do otherwise might shake the patient's faith in the analyst's goodwill and invalidate years of analytic work. The other side considers that to express sympathy might be a mistake—it might prevent the patient from exhibiting satisfaction at the death or, in the future, might inhibit the patient from showing anger toward the analyst. Besides questions of handling the transference, how much interpretation should the analyst provide of the patient's actions or dreams and free associations when they do come up? To interpret too much (as Freud apparently did) is to have the interpretation fall on deaf ears, with a consequent loss of faith in the analyst, or to arouse anxiety in the patient concerning material he is not ready to confront—to interpret too little is to let significant material go by unnoted and hence prolong the analysis unnecessarily. The ideal, of course, is when the patient makes the significant interpretation him- or herself. The course of each psychoanalysis is a very individual matter and analysts may change their approach as years go by to achieve better results.

How capable is psychoanalysis in effecting a desired change? Freud gave his appraisal in one of his last works, "Analysis Terminable and Interminable," written in 1937. Noting how psychoanalysis was more

and more taking on the task of analyzing an individual's entire personality and the difficulties of this kind of analysis, he wrote:

> One has the impression that one ought not to be surprised if it
> should turn out in the end that the difference between a person
> who has not been analyzed and the behavior of a person after he
> has been analyzed is not so thoroughgoing as we aim at making it
> and as we expect and maintain it to be.

The objective of psychoanalysis is long-lasting change in personality.
It is an arduous task that can in some cases be accomplished; it depends
very much on the individual patient and the psychoanalyst. Changes
may often be modest, as intimated by Freud, but such modest changes
occurring at an appropriate time of life have proved to be of considerable benefit to individuals.

Perhaps more important philosophically is Freud's view that psychoanalysis might allow for an understanding of one's own nature. There
seem to be few patients who have managed to free associate to their
dreams who doubt that they are looking at the mysterious undercurrents of their personalities, and there are few analysts who have had
such patients who do not agree. This point was made by long-time
psychoanalyst Bruno Bettelheim in an article in *The New Yorker*. The
title was "Freud and the Soul." Ostensibly, the reason for the article
was to make Freud's work more meaningful by correcting the English
translation of certain of his concepts, among which was the substitu-
tion of the word "soul" for "mind" ("soul" is not meant in the religious
sense but as the basis of the psyche). In essence the article was a
statement of Bettelheim's credo in which he stated what he considered
to be Freud's greatest contribution:

> Freud showed us how the soul could become aware of itself. To
> become acquainted with the lowest depth of the soul—to explore
> whatever personal hell we may suffer from—is not an easy under-
> taking. Freud's findings and even more, the way he presents them
> to us give us the confidence that this demanding and potentially
> dangerous voyage of self-discovery will result in our becoming

more fully human, so that we may no longer be enslaved without knowing it to the dark forces that reside in us. By exploring and understanding the origins and the potency of these forces, we not only become much better able to cope with them but also gain a much deeper and more compassionate understanding of our fellow-man.

Where do we stand in our summary of the findings of psychoanalysis? We return essentially to *The Interpretation of Dreams* and the phenomena of the unconscious, repression, and dream distortion. We add the phenomenon of transference, also widely observed, and the universal agreement among psychoanalysts that early childhood experience is most important in the development of personality.

We now return to the physiology of the brain to look at three specific neural mechanisms. Each contains a particular clue to the psyche. The first is a critical period in the development of the brain early in life. The second and third are neural mechanisms recently found to be operating in the hippocampus and limbic system. These findings, together with those described in the earlier section, Brain, will provide all of the information we need to understand the biology underlying the psychological phenomena I have just described.

Neural Mechanisms

When, as in sleep . . . the activity of the highest sensory centers is uninterfered with by the environment, the very highest nervous arrangements of the highest centers, those in which entirely new organizations can be made, will be in least activity and the next lower nervous arrangements of those centers are left to fight it out among themselves; new combinations arise, the survival of the fittest. . . .

Hughlings Jackson
Croonian Lectures
British Medical Journal
April 12, 1884

Six

CRITICAL PERIOD

After hatching, a duckling, gosling, or chick will follow the first moving object to which it is exposed (under normal circumstances its mother, but under experimental conditions another species such as man or an inanimate object). Once having followed the object, the young bird becomes imprinted on it and will tend to follow the imprinted object or one similar to it for the remainder of its life. The most sensitive period for imprinting is twelve to twenty-four hours after hatching, and it will not occur after thirty-two hours. Ethologists refer to this period as the critical period—a sensitive period for learning during which animals possess special learning capabilities within a specific domain. Beyond this period the ability to learn within this domain ceases, and whatever has been learned constitutes the basis for future behavior.

Recent research has found that a broader critical period exists in the organization of sensory perception and learning in young mammals, including young children. The critical period coincides with the time period during which the neocortex develops anatomically, and it may be related to this development. We will look at three examples of critical period—one in audition, a second in vision, and a third in the organization of a complex behavior, predation in the cat.

The brain of the newborn infant weighs approximately 330 grams (11 ounces). As it matures, the brain increases its weight fourfold. It grows rapidly in size and weight in the first two years of life—its weight triples to about 1,000 grams during this period. It grows substantially to 1,250 grams by the age of seven, then more slowly to 1,350 grams by the age of twelve. It reaches its adult weight of approximately 1,380 grams by the age of fourteen.

All of the neurons of the adult brain are already present in the brain of the infant—the process of cell division (mitosis) is complete before birth. If there is no increase in the number of neurons in the brain, what is responsible for brain growth? The cell bodies of neurons do increase in size somewhat as the brain matures, but most brain growth is accounted for by an increase in the length and branching of the dendrites and axons that connect one neuron to another. There is also an increase in the number of glial cells, cells that are believed to support brain function metabolically.

The growth of dendrites and axons and the development of their interconnections are especially characteristic of neurons in the neocortex. Neocortical neurons are relatively undeveloped at birth. Paralleling the increase in brain weight, there is a rapid maturation of their interconnections during the first two years of life, which continues at a decelerating rate until puberty. This growth is shown on the next two pages.

Is the mammalian brain modified by experience in any irreversible or long-lasting way during this period in which an increasing number of interneuronal connections are being made? That is, is there a critical period for the organization, say, of perception or behavior? The answer is yes, and the first such example we consider has been found in the acquisition of language.

A phoneme is an elemental speech sound from which words are constructed. The word "bet" has three phonemes. The first is the sound made by pronouncing the letter *b* alone (which we may denote as *ba)*, the second is the sound of *e* alone, and the third is the sound of *t.* The words "bet" and "get" are different in their first phonemes but not in their second or third. Similarly the word "debt" differs from "bet" and "get" only in that its first phoneme is *da* rather than *ba* or *ga.* In the late 1940s and early 1950s, two devices came into use in the analysis of language—the sound spectrograph and the speech synthesizer. The sound spectrograph analyzed the frequency components of the sound of phonemes such as *ba, ga,* or *da* and printed them out as a graph of the frequencies present in the sound versus the time during

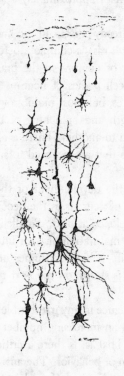 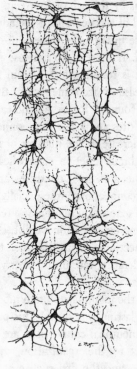

Newborn   3 months

ILLUSTRATION 11

*Neurons of the neocortex are relatively undeveloped at birth. Their dendrites and
axons grow to meet neighboring neurons and form a complex network during the
first two years of life. Shown are neurons from the neocortex of a newborn infant
and infants of three months and six months of age, as well as a child to two years
of age, all of whom died of natural causes unrelated to the brain. The region of
the neocortex from which these sections were prepared is a region of the cortex
which, had these infants lived, would have been involved in the articulation of
speech. Experience influences the connections within the neocortex early in life
during the critical period.*

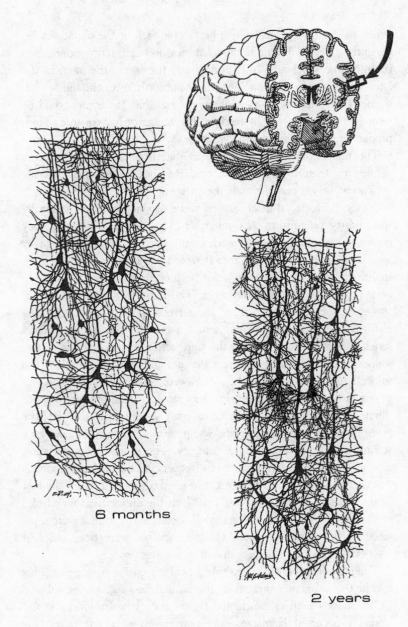

6 months

2 years

which the sound was made. The graphs for each of the phonemes *ba*, *ga*, and *da* were different as the sound was initiated (corresponding to the differences between *b*, *g*, and *d)* and then were the same in the later segments of the phonemes (the *a* portion). With the unique frequency-time patterns of each phoneme available, the sound could be reproduced synthetically by feeding this frequency pattern to a sound-producing device, the speech synthesizer.

The interesting aspect of this was that from the sound patterns defined by their frequency-time characteristics, intermediate sounds could now be generated. From the spectrographs of *ba*, *da*, and *ga*, a series of thirteen artificial sounds were produced, which gradually spanned the range from *ba* through *da* to *ga*. As far as the frequency components were concerned, each of the thirteen sounds was equally spaced from its neighbors. Subjects were then asked to identify these sounds as they were played in order from *ba* to *ga*. There appeared to be abrupt perceptual discontinuities. The frequency changes between successive sounds were equal but the subjects did not detect a gradual change. The first series of four sounds were heard as *ba*, the second series of four or five as *da* and the third series as *ga*. Only one or two sounds at the boundaries between *ba*, *da*, and *ga* were found by the subjects to be ambiguous—the others were considered clear examples of one of the three phonemes. Further, subjects could not discriminate differences of sound within a given category. A sound within one of the given phonetic categories (say *da)* was presented and was followed by a second sound within the same category. The sounds were different, separated by a definite increment in frequency. One of the two sounds was then repeated, and the subjects were asked to say if it was the first or the second. The subjects could not hear the difference; their choice was no better than a random guess. However, if the sounds were separated by the same increment of frequency but were from different phonetic categories, the discrimination was immediate.

The phenomenon was called categorical perception. It occurred only within the phonemes present in the natural language of the subject. Other sounds such as protracted steady state vowels, which do not normally occur in language, were not perceived categorically. Like many other nonspeech sounds, there was continuous perception in that steady state vowel sounds differing by small changes in frequency could be discriminated from one another.

The categories of phonemic perception were strongly dependent on the language heard by the subjects in their childhood. The sounds *l* and *r* do not occur in the Japanese language. The difficulty experienced by Japanese in using these sounds in speaking English is well known. Tests of the type described above indicated that if Japanese was the only language heard during childhood, a subject did not hear *l* and *r* categorically. It appeared that with early exposure to English, the brain became tuned to the phonetic categories used in English words and thus allowed the listener to distinguish clearly one phoneme from another despite the variability encountered in normal speech. To Japanese listeners there was a large area of ambiguity. Extremes in *l* and *r* pronunciation could be identified but many intermediate pronunciations could not, so Japanese listeners frequently did not hear *l* and *r* in spoken English. There are a number of other instances of phonemic contrasts in one language that do not exist in another. For example, the Thai language contains certain phonemes which are not present in English, and consequently English-speaking people have considerable difficulty with Thai.

The ontogenetic development of categorical perception was studied in two- to three-month-old infants. The technique was to present to the infant a graded series of phonetic sounds and to make continuous measurements of either its heart rate or its rate of sucking on a nipple. As the infant was habituated to a given sound, its heart or sucking rate became steady—then the next sound, slightly different in frequency pattern was presented and then the next. At a certain point in the sequence, the infant showed a sudden change in heart or sucking rate. Presumably it was alerted by what it sensed as a new category of sound. Experiments of this type indicated that infants hear categorically in certain phonemic dimensions. However, the categories thus determined did not correspond to the language in the environment but appeared to be universal. This suggested the existence of an inborn perceptual mechanism, ready to be modified so as to perceive optimally the particular phonemes heard by a child during the first few years of life.

A critical period was found for the development of phonemic categories. Normal language development in infants proceeds from babbling
to words during the period of four months to two years of age. Two-
year-olds can identify and clearly use the perceptual categories of the
language to which they have been exposed. The child is in a natural
state for learning languages at this time and for several years thereafter.
If exposed to several languages, perceptual categories are built up for
each, and even if exposure to a given language is discontinued, learning
the language later is greatly facilitated and the person can turn from
one language to another without confusion or accent. A foreign accent
in a language is an indication that the phonemic modules formed in
early childhood in the speaker are different from those of the language
now being spoken. The phonemic categories established early in life are
persistent. Foreign accents cannot be overcome easily after puberty.

Beyond the development of phonemic categories, there is a critical
period for the acquisition of language itself. While the learning of a
second language is a seemingly natural process in childhood, it is laborious after puberty. Eric Lenneberg of Harvard Medical School, who
studied the acquisition of language extensively, set the critical period
for learning language—that is, the period during which the neural basis
for language is formed and in a sense solidified—at two to twelve years
of age. Below the age of two, the neocortex is insufficiently mature to
sustain the organization of language, and beyond twelve, any new learning of language that takes place appears to be based in a different and
less efficient neural mechanism than the mechanism that underlies
learning during the critical period.

What is the function of categorical perception? How did it evolve
and what is its neural substrate? The ability of the brain to construct
acoustic categories tuned to the phonemes heard early in life constitutes the basis of word perception and language. The neural mechanism underlying this effect may have arisen along with language in
man. Language, made possible by the evolutionary growth of the neocortex, clearly provided man with a selective advantage in survival. Or
categorical perception may have first appeared in an animal ancestral to
man, in which the ability to perceive sounds in the habitat categorically
(say calls of warning from fellow creatures) provided the animal a simi-

lar selective advantage. As for the neural substrate, we will postpone this discussion until the other examples of a critical period have been presented.

A second example of a critical period occurs in the visual system. The newborn kitten opens its eyes for the first time at about ten to fourteen days of age. At this time few of the connections within the primary visual cortex that will be present in the adult animal have been formed. For the next several weeks the visual system develops rapidly, and by the age of four weeks most of the adult connections have been made. Also by four weeks of age the kitten shows the first signs of functional visual perception. It can judge its distance from objects in the environment and can place its paws appropriately as it moves among these objects.

The connections being made in the visual cortex during the first four weeks of life are not influenced by visual experience. But then there follows a critical period from the fourth to the twelfth week when visual experience is very important in modifying or refining the connections already made.

David Hubel and Torsten Wiesel, whose work in the cortical columns of the cat and monkey visual cortex I described in Chapter 1, began looking at the connections in the developing brain in 1963. They had established the existence of cortical columns whose neurons responded to lines or edges of a given orientation in an animal's visual field. There were line detectors for horizontal and vertical lines and all oblique angles. These line detectors, they thought, constituted the first of a series of stages by which the brain would ultimately identify complex forms and shapes. There was also an interaction between the two eyes. Neurons detecting a line of a given orientation would do so when seen with either eye but the effects were not equal. Some neurons responded more strongly to an input from the left eye and some more strongly to an input from the right. For a line of a given orientation, these neurons, each dominated by the input from a different eye, lay in neighboring cortical columns called ocular dominance columns. This segregation by ocular dominance, Hubel and Wiesel thought, formed the basis for depth perception.

Having used their experimental procedure to trace the circuits for line detectors and ocular dominance in adult cats, Hubel and Wiesel performed the same experiments in young kittens to see to what extent these circuits operated in these animals with little or no visual experience. They tested an eight-day-old kitten whose eyes had not yet opened and found an organization of the visual cortex similar to the adult cat. There were cells that detected lines of a given orientation, although the orientations were less well defined than in the adult. Since the kitten had no visual experience, the circuits for line detection were apparently determined genetically.

A second kitten was tested at sixteen days of age, but in this case both its eyes were covered with translucent patches from its ninth day. The idea was to allow light to enter but not visual patterns. A third kitten, tested at nineteen days, had one eye covered with a translucent patch from the age of nine days while the other eye was allowed normal vision. A final kitten was tested at twenty days, having had normal vision since its eyes opened at about nine days. All of these manipulations were made to see if these varied types of visual input would alter the developing circuitry of the visual cortex. For example, would lack of patterned input in one eye and diffused light in the other affect the ocular dominance columns? None of these effects occurred. The neural organization set down genetically and observed in the eight-day-old kitten without visual experience was the same in all of the kittens regardless of the varied visual inputs.

Other investigators performed similar experiments and although questions have been raised about the specificity of the line detectors in the newly born kitten, the Hubel and Wiesel results seem reasonably well established. Hubel and Wiesel added further details in later experiments. Although the circuits for line detection are present in very young kittens, the ocular dominance columns are not yet developed. However, by the age of three weeks, ocular dominance columns have been formed, and the kitten possesses a visual system that is organized genetically to accomplish the first steps of feature and depth perception. There then begins a critical period of approximately nine weeks during which visual experience can modify the connections within the system.

Just as they had done in very young kittens, Hubel and Wiesel deprived older kittens of sight in one eye. In these experiments they either used a translucent eye cover or they sutured the lids of one eye closed for varying periods of time—as little as three to four days within the age period of four to twelve weeks. They then removed the translucent cover or opened the lids of the eye. To test the kitten's vision, the eye that had been allowed normal vision was now covered. The kittens behaved as though they were blind in the eye that had been deprived of visual input. To quote from their report:

> As an animal walked about investigating its surroundings the gait was broad-based and hesitant, and the head moved up and down in a peculiar nodding manner. The kittens bumped into large obstacles such as table legs, and even collided with walls, which they tended to follow using their whiskers as a guide. When put onto a table the animals walked off into the air, several times falling awkwardly onto the floor. When an object was moved before the eye there was no hint that it was perceived, and no attempt was made to follow it. As soon as the cover was taken off the left eye (the eye allowed normal visual input) the kitten would behave normally, jump gracefully from the table, skillfully avoiding objects in its way. We concluded that there was a profound, perhaps complete, impairment of vision in the deprived eye of these animals.

The pupillary responses in both eyes were normal—a change had occurred not in the eye but in the visual system of the brain to cause the functional blindness in the eye that had been deprived of visual input. Hubel and Wiesel tested these kittens electrophysiologically using their normal paradigm, presenting lines or edges within the visual field of the kitten of either the left or right eye and measuring the responses of neurons in the primary visual cortex. The results were clear —the connections had changed. Formerly, most neurons responded to an input to either eye although for any given neuron the input from the left or the right eye had a stronger effect. Now almost all of the neurons responded to an input to the normal eye and virtually none to the eye that had been sutured closed or covered with a patch: the connections from the eye that was not allowed to see were no longer operating. And there were no silent areas in the neocortex, which might indicate that cells driven by the eye deprived of vision had died. Rather it seemed that the connections had shifted so that the normal eye had taken over the neurons that were formerly driven by the eye that was closed or covered for a period of time between the third and twelfth weeks.

There was a clear critical period. Beyond the age of twelve weeks, depriving one eye of input had no effect on the visual system. Closing an adult cat's eye for over a year produced no change in the organization of the visual system or in its behavior.

The changes produced during the critical period were irreversible. After dominance was shifted by closing one eye for the first twelve weeks of life, opening the eye for a period of up to five years produced only very limited change in the neural organization back toward normal. There was a particularly sensitive interval in the critical period, the fourth and fifth weeks of life. At this time, three or four days of eye closure led to a sharp change in ocular dominance.

The effect of visual experience during the critical period was not restricted to the organization of the ocular dominance columns. The detectors of oriented lines or edges could be modified as well. In an experiment performed in 1977, Colin Blakemore and Grahame Cooper of the University of Cambridge raised kittens from the age of two weeks to five months in a very selective environment. Most of the time the kittens were in a completely dark room but for five hours each day they were placed on a platform in the center of a tall plastic tube about twenty inches in diameter. On the inside surface of the tube were painted lines of only one orientation, vertical or horizontal. The kittens wore lightweight collars that prevented the animal from seeing its own body, and during the time in the tube, the kittens sat for long periods of time observing the stripes without tilting their heads to either side very much. Thus, in effect, the kitten's entire visual experience was confined to either vertical or horizontal lines.

One kitten was exposed to the horizontal lines and the other to the vertical lines in this experiment. After five months, each kitten behaved as if it could not see lines oriented in the direction in which it had no visual experience. The kitten exposed to horizontal lines ignored a rod that was held vertically and shaken, but immediately ran to the rod and played with it when it was turned horizontally. The opposite was true of the other kitten. The visual cortex of each animal was then explored electrophysiologically for line detectors. Indeed, there were no horizontal line detectors in the kitten that was exposed only to vertical stripes, and this was the reason the kitten could not see the horizontal bar shaken in front of it. Similarly, there were no vertical line detectors in the other kitten. Thus the visual system had been matched to the features of the environment. In later experiments, Blakemore's group verified the effect in other animals and determined that the critical period in kittens for modifying line detectors was the same as for modifying ocular dominance—about three to twelve weeks.

Earlier, in 1970, another experiment had found the same effect. At Stanford University, Helmut Hirsch and Nico Spinelli raised kittens during their critical period wearing goggles in which there were illuminated stripes, horizontal for one eye and vertical for the other. This was the kitten's only visual experience—when not wearing goggles they lived in the dark. At the conclusion of the critical period, neurons in the visual cortex were tested for their responses to lines of various orientations. Neurons responded only to horizontal lines when lines of various orientations were presented to the eye that had seen only horizontal lines—the neurons receiving input from this eye had no detectors for vertical or slanted lines. The opposite was true of the eye that had seen only vertical lines.

The techniques involved in these experiments are complex, and there remain methodological questions regarding the findings just described. However the general result seems clear. Starting with a genetically programmed set of instructions early in life which provide a framework for binocular vision and feature detection, there follows a critical period during which the neural networks underlying vision can be modified by the environment. Beyond the critical period, these changes in neural connectivity no longer occur—the neural networks set up during the critical period become permanent.

There is some indication that this mechanism is present in man. In most cases of astigmatism, blurred vision occurs along orientations close to either the horizontal or the vertical. If the developing visual system is influenced by visual input as animal research has shown, then feature detectors would be lost along the horizontal or vertical direction in which visual input is blurred (just as in Blakemore's kittens the lack of horizontal or vertical visual input eliminated feature detectors sensitive to horizontal or vertical lines). This has been found to be the case. Astigmatism can be fully corrected optically, but in an astigmatic person whose vision was not corrected until the age of six or older, there remains a loss of visual acuity despite full optical correction. And the direction of loss of activity corresponds to the direction in which the early input was blurred by astigmatism.

What is the function of the early flexibility of connections in the normal visual system during the critical period followed by the connections becoming permanent? The neural networks that are responsible for depth perception are extremely complex. Neuroscientists consider it possible that in addition to genetic programming, early experience in seeing objects with both eyes at varying distances results in small modification of the networks, which may be necessary to achieve functional depth perception. It is also possible that the early flexibility of an animal's visual system tunes it optimally to the environment. For example, the feature detectors in the visual systems of animals raised in the jungle or on the plains would, through early experience, become adapted to detect objects best in that particular environment.

The third example of a critical period comes from the work of the German ethologist Paul Leyhausen. The description of the development of predatory behavior that follows is drawn from his book *Cat Behavior*.

Cats do not innately identify any particular species of animal such as a mouse or a bird as natural prey. They learn to select prey, but they are guided by a series of genetically programmed reactions. Thus

Both young and old domestic cats are immensely attracted by rustling and scratching noises and squeaking sounds. Very probably they register on an acoustic IRM [innate releasing mechanism, an innate sensitivity to a particular sensory stimulus, which releases a genetically programmed behavioral response]. What is elicited by this is not prey catching itself but only the appetitive behaviors [appetitive behavior is defined as behavior in search of an appropriate releasing stimulus situation in which a final consummatory act will be performed]. The cat runs more or less straight toward the source of the sound, looking searchingly around at the same time. Crouching, stalking and lying in wait [innate reactions] begin only when the cat sees a movement or if it is already experienced with prey—the prey animal sitting still. However, if it reaches the source of the sound, for example, in deep litter, without anything having appeared, it often feels around with angling movements and either grasps the prey animal with its claws and pulls it into the open, or flushes it thus from cover and chases it optically.

Leyhausen then considers the effect of movement of prey more closely.

Young domestic cats that grow up without having contact with small animals of other species at first regard any other animal as a "fellow cat." If, for instance, a mouse is put with the cat, the mouse remains unnoticed as long as it does not move. If it moves slowly it will be sniffed; but it is chased and pounced on only if it runs quickly away for any distance. Any not-too-large object moving rapidly over the ground elicits the chasing and catching movements, most intensely of all when it runs away from the cat or at right angles to it. In contrast, movement towards the cat causes inexperienced animals to hesitate and, if the size and speed of the object increases, to retreat or even run away. . . . The movement and direction of any movement of a not-too-large object are, therefore, the only factors which innately release a cat's catching actions.

Leyhausen describes how cats kill prey animals by biting the nape of the neck. This innate reaction is very old phylogenetically—cats may have inherited it from their reptilian ancestors. In the cat natural selection also appears to have bred a specific orienting reaction, which directs the attacking bite fairly precisely toward the most fatal spot, the spinal cord. Further, the canine teeth of cats, both in their shape and in their position in the jaws, are well adapted to the "lie" of the muscles, tendons, and ligaments as well as to the directions of the planes of the vertebrae of small prey animals, so that these almost automatically guide at least one of the four penetrating canine teeth to an intervertebral space, thus wedging the vertebrae apart or partially severing the spinal cord.

Leyhausen then considers the role of experiential learning. Besides stimuli that innately release and guide behavior, cats learn by individual experience. They must learn when motionless animals can be considered prey and which animals are to be considered prey at all. They must distinguish prey from members of their own and related species and from superior enemies. And in killing different prey, they must learn how to direct the killing bite effectively for each prey species.

There is an important role for the mother in providing prey-killing experience to her kittens:

When the kittens are about four weeks old, the mother cat begins to carry prey to the nest, but in the beginning she kills it where it is caught and eats it herself in the nest, growling as she does. This spectacle seems at first to frighten the kittens rather than attract them.

In the following weeks the kittens' reaction to the prey animal matures. Thus when the mother brings the first live prey animal along, they have at their disposal a whole arsenal of instinctive movements which are not yet linked up, however, in a chain leading to killing. During play, individual elements may sometimes combine in their later form, e.g., lying in wait with stalking, the stalking run with the pounce, and so on, but at once they separate again and appear singly or in combination with other playful movements, some of which come from other functional contexts than that of prey catching. It also becomes obvious that it is not without reason that the killing bite does not emerge until so late and until the kitten meets its first live prey. If it were otherwise, the kittens would often injure one another while playing at prey-catching among themselves. As they play with the first prey animals, the ordered sequence leading to the killing bite—namely, lying in wait, stalking up, pouncing and seizing—establishes itself gradually, though occasionally it can happen quite suddenly. During this period too, the extent to which the mother cat brings prey to the nest and gives it up to the kittens is gradually stepped up. . . .

The killing bite requires strong additional excitation to elicit it for the first time and this is usually supplied not by the prey itself but by the mother or by the fact that a sibling approaches and is fended off. Thus, when the mother cat lets the live prey run and quickly catches it again, this is not a "demonstration" nor does the kitten learn from "her how it is done." On the contrary, the released prey animal elicits the kitten's prey-catching activity by running away, and its swift recapture by the old cat compels the kitten to be even quicker if it wants to catch the prey before the mother seizes it again. This rivalry provides the additional excitation necessary.

Having related the development of predatory behavior in the kitten, Leyhausen now describes a critical period in that development.

The peak of readiness to kill for the first time which is reached in the ninth and tenth week is maintained for only a short period, and thereafter readiness diminishes again. Kittens whose mother does not bring live prey to them during the critical period between their sixth and about their twentieth week, later either do not kill or else come to do it in a slow, laborious way. . . .

He notes at a later point that the behavioral deficiency in predatory behavior is not completely irreversible. Adult cats without experience can be stimulated to kill prey, but the stimulus required is high.

Finally, Leyhausen describes a second, most important aspect of learning in the cat, its memory for places and its ability to associate past events with them. Thus:

The most important role in the fulfillment of appetence for prey is played by remembrance of locality. As already stated elsewhere, cats possess an exceptionally well-developed memory for places, and after only one positive experience they will often, and repeatedly, seek out a particular place in a room or on a certain piece of land with astonishing precision in order to "look for more," even though many weeks may have elapsed since they last set foot in the area concerned.

These are three instances of a critical period. They all apparently reflect a common phenomenon. The neocortex of the young mammal is in a flexible state. There is a genetically given structure but also coded in the genes is the capability of the neocortex to respond to and be molded in a long-lasting fashion by early experience. This capability allows the formation of neural circuits which are best suited to extract information from the environment and to establish patterns of behavior that are suitable for survival.

The functions of these circuits are diverse—audition, vision, language, strategies of behavior—but the common factor is the neocortex. Audition and vision are mediated by the sensory cortex, language by association cortex on the left side of the brain, and strategies of behavior most probably by the prefrontal cortex. What is the neural mechanism involved? It must be a mechanism that will be plastic and then set. One possibility is that interneuronal connections form (within the neocortex and between the thalamus and the neocortex), which connections are influenced by environmental stimuli during the critical period and then become permanent. This seems to occur in the visual system. There are as yet no data for the rest of the neocortex.

Another possibility involves synaptic facilitation, a process whereby passage of a signal along a particular circuit via particular synapses makes a later passage of a signal along the same circuit easier; therefore a later signal is more likely to flow through this facilitated circuit than through an alternate one. Assume the networks in the thalamus and auditory cortex mediating audition are determined genetically and do not change—that is, there are no new interneuronal circuits formed as in the example above. Hearing a particular phoneme would activate a particular circuit for neuronal signals through this network. With synaptic facilitation operating, hearing the phoneme again would activate this circuit again in preference to other less facilitated ones. This circuit would be activated each time the phoneme is heard, becoming better established with each use, and the brain would use activation of the particular circuit for perception of the phoneme. However, most instances of synaptic facilitation that have been discovered in the brain are not long-lasting. Synaptic facilitation would have to be augmented by a mechanism imparting permanence in order to explain the data. Neuroscientists are seeking such mechanisms in the brain to explain normal learning and memory.*

What clue does the critical period give us to psychological function? In its effect on the prefrontal cortex, we will later find an explanation for the profound influence of early experience on the formation of the unconscious. In addition, Leyhausen's description of predatory behavior in the cat has provided us with an example of the interaction of the innate behavior and learning to which we will refer again. His description also highlighted two of the cats' behaviors, predation and exploration of the environment. We will see in the next chapter how these behaviors are especially significant in this species.

Seven

HIPPOCAMPAL THETA RHYTHM[1]

In the first chapter, we saw how the neocortex analyzes sensory events and got a sense of the intimate association between the hippocampus and the neocortex in processing these events into memory. Anatomical studies suggested that information from primary sensory areas of the neocortex was further processed in associated areas and that the most highly processed information from all of the senses, the information that we recognize as the event itself, converged in a neocortical area called the entorhinal cortex, which then sent a major input to the hippocampus. Further, we saw that H.M. and similar patients could not remember events for more than a short period of time without the hippocampus. In this chapter and the next we will look at the hippocampus more closely and find in its function our last two clues to the neural basis of the psyche.

What kind of neural processing occurs within the hippocampus and what is the interaction of the hippocampus with the neocortex and the rest of the brain? The question is most naturally asked in the context of the awake, attentive states in which we expect an event to be remembered. However, in view of the thought processes that occur during sleep, I will extend the question to the sleep state as well.

John Green and Arnaldo Arduini were studying hippocampal function in the laboratory of neurophysiology at the University of California at Los Angeles in 1953. They had placed electrodes in the hippocam-

---

[1] The reader may find certain passages in this and the chapter that follows somewhat more technical than previous descriptions of the brain. They may be skipped over without undue loss. Summaries at the end of the chapters present the main points.

pus and in the neocortex of rabbits so that they could record electrical activity of both structures simultaneously. They paralyzed the animals with curare, a natural substance extracted from the bark of trees, which blocks the signals from the brain that activate the muscles of the body. They used curare in this experiment because the animals had to remain absolutely stationary, their heads held in a fixed position with a restraining device, so that the delicate electrodes could be moved sequentially to several positions in the hippocampus and other brain structures. However, the animals also had to be awake, unanesthetized, ready to process stimuli as would a normal animal. There was no pain involved since the brain has no pain receptors.

After a time in the restraining device the animals became used to both the restraint and their paralyzed condition. The neocortical EEG showed the rabbits soon becoming drowsy and entering the first stage of slow-wave sleep. The hippocampal record at this time showed a large, irregular signal similar to the large slow waves seen in the neocortical EEG.

The researchers then presented a sensory stimulus to the rabbit—they moved an object within its visual field, sounded a click, presented an odor, or touched the cornea of its eye. The neocortical EEG immediately flattened to the low-level irregular signal normally seen during the alert state. Almost simultaneously the hippocampal record changed to a totally different kind of signal, one that cyclically reversed itself about 6 times per second. This signal, if amplified 100,000 times, would look somewhat like common household AC electric current, except that AC current reverses itself at a faster rate, 60 times per second. Such a smooth, reversing signal is called sinusoidal, since it is the form generated by the mathematical sine function.

Historically, neocortical EEG waves of different frequencies were given different Greek letters as names. The 10 per second waves discovered by Hans Berger were called the alpha rhythm; waves in the neocortex which oscillated at about 4 to 7 times per second were called theta waves, and so when Green and Arduini observed waves at this frequency in the hippocampus, they called these waves theta rhythm. Green and Arduini described the theta rhythm response in the hippocampus as follows:

A train of sinusoidal slow waves of large amplitude and three to six
per second rhythm, often preceded by a primary response of brief
duration, invariably follows olfactory, visual, auditory or tactile
stimulation. . . . In rabbits with chronically implanted electrodes [some animals were tested during normal behavior after
electrodes had been permanently or chronically fixed in the hippo-
campus], slight movement of any object visible to the animal will
evoke a typical train of waves. If the movement is repeated at
intervals the response becomes weaker but reasserts itself immediately when the type of movement is changed. Similar effects have
been obtained by varying auditory stimuli. . . . It seems evident
that the animal adapts in some way to repeated stimuli and is
aroused most effectively by new or strange phenomena.

The paper reporting these results was entitled "Hippocampal Electrical Activity in Arousal." Green and Arduini were the first to study

ILLUSTRATION 12

*Green and Arduini recorded hippocampal and neocortical signals in the drowsy
and in the alert rabbit. The top line is a recording taken in the hippocampus and
the second line a recording in the neocortex. At the beginning of the record the
animal was drowsy and large, irregular waves appeared in both structures. At the
time indicated by the arrow, an olfactory stimulus, the odor of cabbage, was
blown toward the animal's nostrils. The neocortical EEG flattened as is typical
for the alert state while theta rhythm appeared in the hippocampus.*

HIPPOCAMPUS

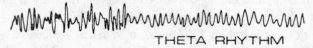

THETA RHYTHM

NEOCORTEX

OLFACTORY STIMULUS

the theta rhythm systematically (its existence had been reported in the 1930s) and had established a correlation of the rhythm with the animal's state of arousal. Other laboratories began to study theta rhythm. The research took two directions. One attempted to define more carefully the behaviors during which the rhythm occurred. The other tried to discover the source of the rhythm and the neural mechanism responsible for generating it. Both sought ultimately to understand theta rhythm's function.

The behavioral aspect of the research turned out to be an intriguing tale that is important in our story.

In view of their observations in the rabbit, it was natural for Green and Arduini to consider that theta rhythm was correlated simply with arousal. But as other behavioral conditions and other species were studied the situation became more complex. Studies were now carried out in rabbits, cats, rats, and other species using electrodes implanted permanently at fixed positions in the hippocampus. Theta rhythm certainly appeared in the rabbit when it was brought to an alert state by a sensory stimulus. It was also present when the animal hopped or walked spontaneously in its environment (in this case a test enclosure) without any externally applied stimulus. However, theta rhythm was not present when the rabbit was awake but had gotten used to its environment, or when it ate or drank or groomed itself.

The behaviors during which theta rhythm appeared in the rat were markedly different. An alerting stimulus was not accompanied by theta rhythm but rather by a low-level irregular hippocampal signal. The stimulus could be minimal (as was effective in the rabbit) or it could be extreme, such as an electric shock delivered to the rat's feet, a loud sound, or an aggressive confrontation with another rat. As long as the rat did not move and remained alert there was no theta rhythm at all. But when the rat explored its environment or moved its head or limbs spontaneously, theta rhythm appeared as it did in the rabbit during similar spontaneous movement. As with the rabbit, during activities such as eating, drinking, grooming, or copulation there was no theta rhythm.

The behaviors for theta rhythm in the cat were different again and somewhat harder to define. There was theta rhythm almost always during voluntary movement although it was usually of low amplitude, and none during automatic behaviors (eating, etc.). The largest amplitudes of theta rhythm occurred during activities that could best be described as predatory—when the cat followed something of interest with its eyes or crouched, ready to spring.

All in all, it looked as though the behaviors during which theta rhythm was generated in the hippocampus in each species were behaviors important for the survival of that species. In the cat these were predation and exploration of the environment (readers will recall Leyhausen's highlighting these behaviors). In the rabbit, escape from predators (based on its sensitivity to the slightest change in its environment), in addition to exploration, generated theta rhythm. In the rat, theta was turned on by exploration itself (the rat is an exploring animal, quickly traversing a new environment, sniffing and moving its vibrissae as it goes, and depending for its survival on the knowledge of its surroundings acquired during exploration). And there was one additional behavioral state in which high amplitude theta rhythm was present continuously in all three species. That state was REM sleep.

Researchers have taken hippocampal recordings in a number of species looking for the presence or absence of theta rhythm. They have found theta rhythm in all lower mammals they have studied, including such diverse species as the tree shrew, dog, squirrel, guinea pig, mouse, mole, and the opossum. There is a well-developed hippocampus in each of these animals—the hippocampus is an old structure phylogenetically, being present in rudimentary form in reptiles—and in each animal theta rhythm appears during some set of behaviors during the waking state (the behaviors associated with theta rhythm have not been defined as closely in these species as in the rabbit, rat, and cat). And in each animal theta rhythm is continuous and prominent during REM sleep. Indeed, nowadays researchers studying lower mammals use the appearance of theta rhythm during sleep as an indication that the animal has entered the REM state. This indicator was especially valuable in the experiment I described earlier in which lesions were made in the brain stems of cats so that motor inhibition was released during REM sleep, allowing cats to act out their dreams. In addition to the other signs of REM sleep such as relaxed nictitating membranes, the presence of continuous theta rhythm in the hippocampus established that the cats were in the REM state and not awake.

Now back to our special animal, the echidna, with its massive prefrontal cortex. The echidna has a normal hippocampus, and Truett Allison noted that there was clear theta rhythm when the animal was awake and burrowing in the shavings of its test cage. He looked carefully for theta rhythm during sleep. There was none, nor were there any indicators of REM sleep, and so he concluded that the REM state did not exist in the echidna. At the other end of the mammalian line, theta rhythm has not yet been found in the hippocampus of man, apes, or monkeys. In all probability there is no such rhythm in any primate.

What is the function of theta rhythm and why, in lower animals, does it appear during important species-specific waking behaviors and, except for the echidna, in REM sleep? What evolutionary change led to its disappearance in man? In the attempt to answer these questions we turn to studies of the mechanisms that generate theta rhythm and for this purpose we must first look at the internal structure of the hippocampus.

The reader will recall my description in the first chapter of the cortical column, the basic processing module of the neocortex. Millions of cortical columns arranged side by side make up the entire neocortex. They act as feature detectors in sensory areas and perform other, as yet unknown, functions in association areas and in the prefrontal cortex. The hippocampus is also made up of elementary processing modules, not columns, but flat segments like poker chips, called lamellae. We have seen that the hippocampus is an elongated, sausagelike structure that fits against the inner wall of the neocortex. The processing modules, the lamellae, are cross-sectional slices of the hippocampus, so that the hippocampus consists of a series of these lamellae, stacked side by side. One can think of the sausage as having been cut into many thin slices which have not been separated.

The processing module of the neocortex, the cortical column, is quite a complicated structure neuroanatomically. It is made up of a number of different types of neurons whose interwiring is just beginning to be unraveled, and it has many entry and exit points through which neuronal signals can pass. The lamella is simpler in its anatomy

—it has only three principal types of neurons, hooked up in a relatively straightforward way. And the flow of information through the lamella, the stages of processing through which an incoming signal passes as it proceeds through the lamella, is reasonably well understood.

As I described in Chapter 1, the major input to the hippocampus comes from a portion of the neocortex called the entorhinal cortex, in which sensory information has received its most refined analysis. Neural signals carrying this information constitute the input to the lamella and reach the first of the three principal cell types in the lamella. Some processing of the incoming information, the logic of which is unknown, occurs at this first stage, and the signal is then transmitted to a second stage where further processing is performed. Finally, the signal is passed to the third main set of neurons, where a third stage of processing is carried out.*

As was seen in Chapter 1, information from the hippocampus is directed to a number of other brain structures in the limbic system. It also returns to the neocortex without passing through the limbic system, so that in effect, the neocortex feeds information to the hippocampus, and the hippocampus then returns the processed information to the neocortex. Somehow within this loop—neocortex to hippocampus to neocortex—and within the circuit from neocortex to hippocampus to limbic system (with an ultimate return to the neocortex), sensory information, analyzed in various sensory centers of the neocortex, is brought together to record an event and remember it. I will return to this circuitry in the next chapter. The point I want to make here is that theta rhythm has been found to be produced within two of the three main groups of neurons in the hippocampus and, as we shall see, has an important influence on the information processing that goes on in that structure.

What are the neurophysiological mechanisms responsible for theta rhythm? In the second chapter, in connection with the alpha rhythm, I suggested that a clear cyclic wave recorded by an EEG electrode probably reflects the synchronous electrical activity of a population of neurons. This electrical activity in the generating neurons must be considerably greater than any nonsynchronous activity of other neurons close to the electrode, or the recorded signal would be mixed at best. Early investigators surmised that such synchronous activity must be responsible for the theta rhythm, and further, that the rhythm was produced in the hippocampus, because the rhythm was strongest when the recording electrode was placed in that structure. They were correct, but the task of identifying the actual generating neurons took some time.

Identifying the cells which produce a rhythm such as the alpha and theta rhythms cannot be done with a scalp electrode. It is best accomplished by passing a recording electrode step by step through the brain. As the electrode approaches the generating neurons, the amplitude of the rhythmic signal will increase, and it will decrease as the electrode passes the neuron population. There are other electrical signs that may also aid in identifying the generator cells. Such studies with penetrating electrodes have not been successfully carried out for the alpha rhythm or for the mixed rhythms that occur during slow-wave sleep, so the sources of these signals remain a mystery. But such studies were performed in the hippocampus soon after the discovery of the theta rhythm by Green and several of his colleagues. They watched the theta rhythm as they lowered an electrode step by step through the hippocampus of rabbits paralyzed by curare. Because of the position of the hippocampus in the rabbit brain, the first cells they encountered were the neurons constituting the third (and last) stage of the circuit within the lamella. The theta rhythm was greatest there, and on the basis of this and other electrical signs, they concluded that theta rhythm was produced by the electrical currents flowing cyclically in these cells. They did not find theta rhythm in the first and second stage neurons of the hippocampal circuit.

Other neurophysiologists were able to position very fine electrodes directly into the bodies of these third-stage neurons, a technique known as intracellular recording, and measured the currents within these cells. Indeed currents were flowing in these neurons, changing their direction about 6 times per second. The result of this constantly changing current was an unusual mode of neural function. Signals were arriving at this third stage of the hippocampal circuit from the neocortex, having been transmitted through the first two stages. If the animal was engaged in an activity during which theta rhythm was being generated in the neurons of this stage, the rhythm determined whether or not the signal passed through the third stage. Theta rhythm was modulating the signals passing through the hippocampus.* I will return to the possible meaning of this kind of neural processing and other aspects of theta rhythm generation in a moment, but I want now to follow the story in a somewhat different direction.

My own interest in theta rhythm began in 1972 and revolved around the unusual behavioral properties of the rhythm—its occurrence during species-specific waking activities and REM sleep—and the neural process that might be going on in the hippocampus during these activities. Theta rhythm was present during several activities in each animal. Were the generating neurons in the three-stage chain the same during all of these behaviors suggesting that the same neural process was occurring in the hippocampus during each of them? I studied unanesthetized rats and rabbits. The animals were free to move within a test enclosure, to explore, eat, drink, groom, and sleep. They were also presented with sensory stimuli. Movable electrodes were advanced step by step through the hippocampus to determine the source of theta rhythm, just as had been done by Green and associates in the curarized rabbit. It will be recalled that in the rat, theta rhythm occurred during one waking activity—spontaneous or voluntary movement—and also during REM sleep. The neurons generating theta rhythm were found to be the same in both activities. This was true in the rabbit as well. When a rabbit was either presented with a sensory stimulus, moved spontaneously, or was in REM sleep, the same neurons were being activated to generate theta rhythm.

But the neurons generating theta rhythm were not merely the neurons in the third stage of the three-stage circuit. The neurons of the first stage of the circuit were also generating the rhythm. In the earlier work of Green and associates the use of curare had apparently masked the generator. So in both rats and rabbits (and this was later confirmed in cats) signals from the neocortex were modified by theta rhythm at two stages of the basic circuit within the lamella, and this process was operative during particular waking behaviors important for the survival of each species and during REM sleep. In 1980 studies performed on rats in the laboratory of James Ranck, Jr., professor of physiology at the Downstate Medical Center in New York, revealed yet a third set of neurons within the neocortex itself (in the entorhinal cortex) in which theta rhythm was generated, again during the same behaviors. In sum, it appeared as though the entire cortical-hippocampal circuit was being rhythmically modulated. And indeed when one records the firing pattern of individual neurons in the hippocampus when an animal is exploring, in REM sleep or in any other activity in which theta rhythm is present in the hippocampus, many of them are found to fire in synchrony with the theta rhythm.

The circuitry that generates theta rhythm begins in the lower brain, the brain stem. Some comment about the brain stem is in order. The brain stem along with two other structures, the cerebellum and the basal ganglia (which are involved with body movement), constitute virtually the entire brain in reptiles, serving to govern all of their life-sustaining processes such as respiration, heart rate, feeding, sexual activity, and the simple repertoire of behaviors, largely genetically determined, by which reptiles survive. Other brain structures evolved later, and with the mammals came the limbic system and the neocortex. The way of evolution was to have these new parts of the brain exert control over the brain stem—to integrate the brain stem into the newer brain so that directions for behavior came from the newer structures above. And because these directions were "intelligently" produced, the behaviors were now flexible, suited to environmental situation by learning. Nevertheless, the most basic life-sustaining processes such as respiration, heart rate, and in mammals the sleep-waking cycle, remained in the control of the brain stem. Thus, when one finds a function controlled from the brain stem, one considers it to be an important basic biological function. This is the case with theta rhythm, which is initiated by brain-stem action.

The neural circuits by which the brain stem produces theta rhythm in the hippocampus are poorly understood. It involves a complicated pathway with several relay stations, the last of which is in a part of the limbic system called the septum. Here the rhythmic cyclic activity begins and is then translated into theta rhythm in the hippocampus. Whatever the mechanism, initiating theta rhythm appears to be genetically programmed so that the rhythm is generated during a particular set of waking activities in each species—and during REM sleep in all.*

What is the function of theta rhythm? It has not been determined, but there are some suggestive findings. I noted that rats are exploring animals. In a new environment they sniff and move their vibrissae back and forth as they walk and poke their heads into corners or rear up to view their surroundings. It has been found that the frequency of this rhythmic cyclic inhalation and vibrissae movement is the same as the theta rhythm.* One may speculate that in animals such as the rat which make great use of the sense of smell it is important that all sensory information, touch sensations from the vibrissae, vision, and hearing are coordinated with the cyclic inhalation of odors. In this way the entorhinal cortex, hippocampus, and the rest of the limbic system can process all sensory input along with smell—an event is linked to its odor. Theta rhythm would then be the neural mechanism for processing sensory information in coordinated short cyclic bursts.

Hippocampal theta rhythm has not been found in monkeys, apes, or man although occasional reports of theta rhythm in man have appeared (it must be said that the search for theta rhythm in primates has not been as thorough as that in lower mammals). If indeed there is no theta rhythm in primates, one would imagine that somewhere along the evolutionary line which gave rise to primates, this cyclic mode of processing sensory information disappeared much as tactile vibrissae did.

Let us summarize. Hippocampal theta rhythm is an indicator of a special type of information processing in the hippocampus. Its mechanism is not completely understood, but it seems to play a role in synchronizing sensory information in lower mammals. The important point to us is the selection of activities in which it occurs. In the waking state, these are species-specific behaviors, basic to the survival of each species. Thus in the rat, theta rhythm occurs during exploration (as it does in the rabbit and cat). In the rabbit it also appears in response to any movement in the environment of which the rabbit must be aware if it is to escape from predators, and in the cat, theta rhythm is most prominent when the cat is tracking prey. The same neurons in the hippocampus are performing the same process characterized by theta rhythm during one other behavioral state, REM sleep, when there is no sensory input from the outside world; it is as if certain information gathered during the day, information associated with survival behaviors, was being dealt with again by structures in which theta rhythm is generated: the entorhinal cortex and the hippocampus.

What connection does all this have to our understanding the psyche? I will suggest that in theta rhythm we have a clue to the evolutionary origin of dreaming in man and to the function of dreams.

Eight

NEURONAL GATING IN THE HIPPOCAMPUS

The limbic system is the central core processor of the brain, in which memory and emotion are integrated, and the hippocampus is its gateway. Information from the neocortex is processed by the hippocampus, then transmitted to limbic system components. As I mentioned earlier, the complexities of limbic system function are largely unexplored; this research is at the frontier of neuroscience. But research has yielded one experimental finding about the inner workings of the limbic system—neuronal gating in the hippocampus—and this constitutes the last clue in the trail we have been following.

This particular story begins with the monoamines. The monoamines are a special class of neurotransmitters used by three systems in the brain. Each system consists of a small number of neurons in the brain stem which send their axons to many brain regions. Prominent among these regions is the limbic system. Each of the monoamine systems arises in a different location in the brain stem, and each has its own set of targets in the brain (although most target areas receive inputs from more than one system). Each uses its own monoamine transmitter, either norepinephrine, serotonin, or dopamine. Compared to other neural systems in the brain, the monoamine systems are unique in several ways. Their neurons have very thin axons, which conduct action potentials from the cell body to target areas more slowly than do most other axons in the brain. In fact, these axons are so thin that they were not detected until the 1960s when Swedish anatomists introduced a technique that allowed them to be visualized. The cells themselves fire at slow rates. At the ends of the axons, the monoamine transmitters seem not to act as other transmitters do, producing action potentials in target cells, but rather they appear to modulate the effect produced by other neurons that also impinge on these same target cells (this point will be illustrated in the hippocampus later).

The norepinephrine system serves as an example. Floyd Bloom, professor of neurobiology at the Salk Institute in La Jolla, California, and his associates have done extensive research on this system. There are approximately 5,000 norepinephrine-containing cells in the brain stem of a rat on each side of its brain. About one third of these lie in a cluster of cells called the locus coeruleus, and these cells project to the limbic system and the neocortex. The locus coeruleus is present in all mammals from echidna to man. Axons of locus coeruleus cells terminate in many limbic system structures, hippocampus and amygdala among them, as well as in the neocortex, and the endings are in specific places in each structure. Bloom and his colleagues have measured the firing rate of these cells in freely moving rats and monkeys. The cells are almost totally silent during REM sleep, fire slowly during slow-wave sleep, and fire at their maximum rate, still only about four or five times a second, when the animal is alert, especially when alerted from sleep.

The function of the norepinephrine system has not been clearly established despite intensive investigation, but Bloom suggests that it may be to prepare the brain to deal most effectively with the environmental situation which has brought the animal to an alert state. He suggests that sensory neurons in the neocortex may decrease their random firing and respond more strongly to outside sensory stimuli as a result of the increased input from norepinephrine neurons during the alert state. This would be an appropriate tuning or modulation of the sensory systems as the animal awakes from sleep or is otherwise roused into an alert state and then must react to stimuli in the environment.

The norepinephrine, serotonin, and dopamine systems send widespread inputs to the limbic system. What these neurotransmitters do in the limbic system is a most interesting question in its own right, and I will return to it later, but it assumes added significance when one realizes that psychoactive drugs, and drugs that ameliorate the symptoms of depression and schizophrenia, act on precisely these three neurotransmitters.

That this is so was discovered accidentally. The first finding concerned depression. In 1952 physicians observed that patients being treated for tubercular pneumonia with the drug isoniazid displayed a distinct elevation of mood. As a result of this finding, depressed patients were soon afterward treated experimentally with iproniazid, a drug closely related to isoniazid but with less dangerous side effects. Iproniazid proved to have clear antidepressive and euphoriant properties. It has since been shown that iproniazid works in this way: an action potential, after traveling along an axon, reaches the synapse at the end of the axon and here releases a small amount of a neurotransmitter, in the case of a monoamine neuron either norepinephrine, serotonin, or dopamine. The transmitter diffuses across the very narrow synaptic cleft to affect the target neuron. Excess neurotransmitter in the synaptic cleft is now rapidly removed to prepare the system for the transmission of the next action potential. The excess transmitter is removed by two means. Either it is broken down to inactive components within the cleft, or it is sucked back into the synaptic ending from which it was released, here to be broken down in the case of monoamine transmitters by the enzyme monoamine oxidase. The action of iproniazid is to inhibit monoamine oxidase. This has the effect of inhibiting the breakdown of norepinephrine and serotonin, thus raising the brain levels of these neurotransmitters. The antidepressant properties of iproniazid and other drugs that inhibit monoamine oxidase are believed to result from these increased levels.

Starting in 1957, antidepressant drugs of a second class, the tricyclic antidepressants, were formulated. They have proved to be more effective in the treatment of depression than the monoamine oxidase inhibitors; they are accompanied by fewer side effects, and consequently are in widespread use today. These drugs also increase the effective levels of norepinephrine and serotonin in the brain, in this case by blocking the normal reuptake into the synaptic ending of the norepinephrine or serotonin that has been released into the synaptic cleft. Thus both classes of drugs that have clinical antidepressant properties appear to exert their effects via the norepinephrine and serotonin systems.

About the same year that physicians first noted the action of isonia-zid, another chance observation led to the formulation of the drugs that ameliorate the symptoms of schizophrenia, the so-called major tranquilizers or neuroleptics. A drug, chlorpromazine, had been synthe-sized as a sedative to use in combination with anesthetic agents. Chlor-promazine did not disturb a patient's conscious awareness, yet the pa-tient became completely uninterested in his or her surroundings. It appeared to early observers to induce a state resembling that produced surgically by frontal lobotomy. Chlorpromazine and other drugs of its class, the phenothiazines, were soon in extensive psychiatric use in the treatment of schizophrenia. The phenothiazines are believed to exert their effects via the norepinephrine and dopamine systems. A second and more recently developed set of compounds, the butyrophenones, the main representative of which is the drug haloperidol, are also effec-tive antipsychotic agents and are also believed to act via the monoamines. In this case the main action appears to be on dopamine while norepinephrine is affected to a lesser extent. In all, there is a close relationship between the monamine neurotransmitters and particular states of mental illness.

The mechanisms of action of the antidepressant and neuroleptic drugs are known to some extent on the neuronal level, but there are many unanswered questions. For example, researchers have found in experiments on animals that the action of the antidepressant com-pounds on neurons is immediate, but when these drugs are taken by patients, they take days or weeks to affect their mental state. One major problem is that the specific neural circuits in which these drugs act to produce their clinical effects are not known. Norepinephrine, serotonin, and dopamine send their axons to many parts of the brain. Which of these are involved? As I mentioned previously, it is generally considered that these drugs may act in the limbic system to produce their effects because of the association of this system with memory and emotion, but there is no evidence that this is so. We do not have sufficient understanding of those neuronal systems that deal with cogni-tion, affect, and memory to comprehend the action of the psychoactive drugs. However, let us leave these matters for the present and return to the hippocampus and the main point of this chapter.

The reader will recall from the last chapter that the presence of theta rhythm in the hippocampus was believed to reflect a particular type of neural processing that involved cyclic modulation of input signals. This occurred only during certain specific activities, suggesting that the hippocampus was changing its mode of information processing when behavior changed. A second set of data carried the same implication. As already described, norepinephrine neurons in locus coeruleus provide a broad input to the hippocampus, and these neurons have different firing rates during different activities—the cells fire more rapidly during the alert state than during sleep. Therefore, more norepinephrine is presumably released in the hippocampus during the alert state than during sleep, and so whatever the effect norepinephrine may have on neural processing in the hippocampus, it will presumably be greatest when the animal is alert, and it will be reduced or absent when the animal is asleep. Thus, neural processing in the hippocampus may be expected to change with changes in behavior on this account. The serotonin cells of the lower brain stem also send inputs to the hippocampus and although the firing rate of these cells during different activities is not well established, it would not be surprising if they also provided a behaviorally dependent influence on hippocampal function.

These data on theta rhythm and monoamine input to the hippocampus led me and a colleague, Charles Abzug, in 1978, to undertake an experiment to test neural processing in the primary three-stage hippocampal circuit during various behavioral states. The experiment was conducted in freely moving rats. I mentioned earlier that the basic hippocampal circuit, contained within the lamella, consists of three stages of processing. This is best seen in the illustration on page 199.

The input signal to the lamella comes from the entorhinal cortex. It first passes through two stages of processing (1 and 2). There is an output from the second stage (output 1) by which the processed signal is passed on to particular structures of the limbic system. The signal also continues within the lamella to the third and final processing stage (3), from which a second output (output 2) carries the signal to the other limbic structures. Each of the two outputs reaches separate limbic system targets so that the flow of information is quite specific—information which has passed through two stages of processing is transmitted to certain limbic structures, information which has undergone three stages of processing is transmitted to others.

The paths of information flow may actually be traced in the brain. A stimulating electrode can be placed in the pathway that leads from the neocortex to the hippocampus. An electrical pulse applied to this pathway then mimics the normally occurring signal from the neocortex; this results in simultaneous action potentials in a number of the input axons to the first stage of the hippocampal circuit. Recording electrodes placed in each of the major cell groups in the lamella can then be used to monitor the resultant firing of each of these groups. The first cell group responds a few thousandths of a second after the input pulse is applied. The second group fires a few thousandths of a second later, and a third group of cells a few thousandths of a second later still. The firing of a particular cell group indicates that the input signal has been processed and transmitted through that particular stage of the circuit.*

We tested animals in four behavioral states, two waking states and the two states of sleep. The waking states were a still-alert condition in which the rat was brought to attention by some stimulus and was not moving, and exploration in which the animal moved about in its cage; the sleeping states were slow-wave sleep and REM sleep. In each of the four behavioral conditions, we sent signal pulses into the hippocampus, through the three-stage chain, and the responses of neurons were recorded at each stage of the circuit. The results showed a dramatic change in the flow of neural signals through the three-stage chain depending on the activity of the animal.

As an example, let us examine what occurred at the third and last stage of processing during the various behavioral states. An input pulse was applied while the rat was in slow-wave sleep. The animal was not disturbed since the pulse did not affect any sensory or motor part of the brain. A recording of the third-stage neurons showed that large numbers of them fired in response to the input. This indicated that the signal had been transmitted through this stage, having previously passed through the first two stages.

The rat then entered REM sleep. The same strength pulse was applied to the input pathway, but there was very little firing of third-stage neurons. When the animal returned to slow-wave sleep, the re-

ILLUSTRATION 13

Shown in the lower part of the figure is the lamella, a cross-sectional slice of the hippocampus which contains the basic three-stage hippocampal circuit. The input to the circuit is from the entorhinal cortex, which receives highly analyzed information from sensory areas of the neocortex. This information is processed and transmitted through a first and then a second stage of the circuit (1 and 2). The first output of the circuit to other structures of the limbic system comes from the second stage (output 1). Information is further processed at a third stage of the circuit (3). A second output of the hippocampus to limbic areas, as well as back to entorhinal cortex, arises at this point (output 2). The pattern of neuronal transmission from entorhinal cortex through the three-stage circuit to its various target areas depends on the behavioral state of the animal.

sponse was large again. Therefore, the neural signal passed through the entire three-stage circuit and was transmitted to limbic system targets via the output from this stage during slow-wave sleep, but the signal was not transmitted during REM sleep. If one imagines a gate at the third-stage junction of the chain, then it was open during slow-wave sleep and closed during REM sleep. (The term "gate" is used in electronic circuitry in analogy with its common meaning. An open gate lets a signal pass through a junction while a closed gate shuts it off or restricts it. Neurophysiologists have extended the metaphor to neural circuits.) In addition, this neural gate was also found to be closed during the two waking states in which the rat was tested, which means the gate remained open only during slow-wave sleep.

Similar gating effects were found at each stage of the three-stage chain so that, depending on the rat's activity, a signal from the neocortex would sometimes pass freely through the entire circuit and be transmitted by second and third stage output axons to all limbic target areas, while at other times it would be preferentially transmitted through the second-stage axons to a subset of these targets (the condition in which the neural gate at stage three was closed), and at still other times it would be restricted in transmission at the first stage of the circuit.

In studying the brain, neuroscientists are used to thinking in terms of fixed anatomical circuits with information being passed along these circuits in the form of a sequence of action potentials. The neural gating phenomenon represents, in effect, a switching of these circuits

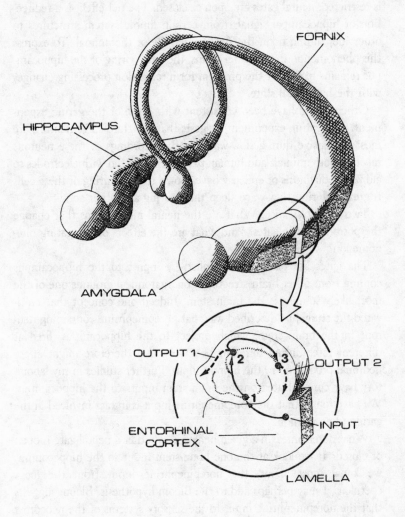

FORNIX

HIPPOCAMPUS

AMYGDALA

OUTPUT 1

2

3

OUTPUT 2

1

INPUT

ENTORHINAL
CORTEX

LAMELLA

within the hippocampus. The circuits do not change their connections but during particular activities information flow along certain pathways is restricted; neural gates are open or closed. The net effect is a redirection of hippocampal signals from certain limbic system structures to others depending upon the state of activity of the animal. To express this phenomenon in computer terms, the hard wiring of the hippocampus remains fixed, but the program for information processing changes with the behavioral state.

Other results have been consistent with those of the gating experiment. The gating experiment suggests that the third-stage neurons are most responsive during slow-wave sleep. Recordings of these neurons taken in both animals and human patients implanted with electrodes to aid in the diagnosis of epilepsy have shown that the firing of these cells is greater during slow-wave sleep than during any other activity.

Two questions arise. What are the neural mechanisms that change the position of the gates? And what are the effects of the gating phenomenon?

The gates are probably controlled by inputs to the hippocampus coming from other brain structures; on anatomical grounds one of the most likely sources is the brain stem. Indeed one concept that motivated the study just described was that norepinephrine containing neurons in the brain stem, which project to the hippocampus, fired at different rates during different behaviors, and therefore might affect neuronal processing in the hippocampus. Further studies in my laboratory have concentrated on the brain stem inputs to the hippocampus. We have found that the norepinephrine input is in fact involved in the gating phenomenon.*

What determines, in a given behavior, whether a neural gate is open or closed? If we look at the one brain-stem input to the hippocampus we know most about, the norepinephrine input from the locus coeruleus, I may perhaps add to the Bloom hypothesis. Bloom suggests that the norepinephrine input to the sensory systems of the neocortex tunes these systems in a manner appropriate to the alert state. That is, the norepinephrine input produces more efficient processing of sensory information at a time when this information is of special importance to the animal, when a stimulus in the environment has brought the animal to a vigilant state, ready to react. Similarly, I would hypothesize that via several brain-stem inputs, the norepinephrine input among them, hippocampal circuitry is functionally modified during certain activity states in a manner appropriate to these activities, so that a specific information processing function is performed during these states.

What is this information processing function? What is the actual effect produced by the changing states of the neural gates? This raises the question of the function of the hippocampus itself. If the lamellae are processing modules in the hippocampus as cortical columns are believed to be in the neocortex, then what is the process? Looking for the moment at the interaction of the hippocampus with the neocortex, we saw from H.M.—and researchers believe from many experiments in animals—that the process here relates to memory. If an event at a given moment consists of information from several sensory modalities detected and analyzed by the neocortex, then is the hippocampus instrumental in organizing and recalling the time sequence of instantaneous, discrete events to allow the recollection of an event in time? Or is the hippocampus involved at an earlier stage, helping in the recall of a memory by connecting together the various sensory impressions that made up the event of the moment? And what of the processes occurring in the limbic system as a whole?

The answers to these questions are not known. A group of hippocampal neuroscientists around the world, myself among them, are attempting to discover them. But what we do know about neuronal gating—the fact that changes in behavior are accompanied by changes in neuronal transmission through the hippocampus—yields another clue important to our hypothesis.

There is one other aspect of hippocampal function that we must consider for which some of the complex neural machinery of the hippocampus and limbic system is perhaps required. It is the unusual matter (discussed in the first chapter) of the three-year period during which the hippocampus is apparently involved in some process whereby a memory is consolidated or reorganized, such that after this time the hippocampus itself is no longer required for the memory's retrieval.

This phenomenon is completely mysterious; however in the last section of this book I offer some possible explanations.

To recapitulate, the hippocampus plays a central role in the limbic system, processing and distributing neocortical information to other limbic system structures. Like circuitry in the rest of the brain, one thinks of hippocampal circuits as fixed, transmitting information along its various pathways in the form of changing patterns of action potentials. But we have discovered an unusual phenomenon, neuronal gating. As an animal's behavioral state changes—waking, slow-wave, REM sleep—influences from the brain stem (and perhaps other sources) affect the hippocampal circuits. They do not change anatomically, but they do change functionally, routing information through the hippocampus differently depending upon behavior. Thus, there is a change of information processing as the animal proceeds cyclically through its normal sequence of waking and sleeping.

What is the purpose of this change of information processing? I will suggest that it underlies the mental processes that sleep research has revealed—dreaming being the foremost among them—and that it constitutes the neural substrate for a brain mechanism evolved early in the history of mammals, a mechanism that constitutes what Freud saw as the unconscious.

All of the evidence is now in: We have seen the machinery of the brain that deals with perception, memory, emotion, sleep, and early development, and the psychological phenomena, that is, the unconscious and its various ramifications. In the next section, we will find that the data from the brain are consistent with the psychological phenomena and, according to my hypothesis, provide an understanding of their biological origin.

Hypothesis

The distant goal to which these investigations lead is a phylogeny of the mind, which, like the body, has attained its present form through endless transformations.

C. G. Jung
Critique of Psychoanalysis

Nine

HYPOTHESIS

I now present to the reader my hypothesis—my idea of what the brain mechanisms may be that underlie unconscious mental processes. The theory is speculative, but since it is based on the physiology of the brain, I expect that ultimately it will be testable by neuroscientific methods and thus subject to correction or refutation.

The key is evolution—the evolution of the dreaming state. We turn back some 180 million years to the time when the monotremes, the echidna among them, were nature's only mammals—the first offshoot of the reptilian species. (You will recall that the monotremes were mammals by virtue of the fact that they were warm-blooded, had hair and four-chambered hearts, and nursed their young with milk. They differed from later marsupial and placental mammals in that, like reptiles, they hatched their young from eggs.) We noted that the echidna was exceptional because of its brain—it had a huge, convoluted prefrontal cortex. And it was unusual in one other respect; it had no REM sleep. (Neither was there REM sleep in reptiles. This stage of sleep had not yet evolved.) Evolution proceeded, and marsupial and placental mammals arose from a line divergent from the monotremes. There were animals among them that were insectivores like the echidna and were quite similar to the echidna in habits and capabilities. But in none of these animals was there anything but a very small prefrontal cortex, and in all of them, as well as in all succeeding mammals, there was REM sleep.

I suggest that with the marsupials and the placentals, nature arrived at a particular solution to a basic problem of the mammalian state—

how to integrate experience over time, that is, how to construct or modify neural circuits to guide future behavior. This integrative process is learning, a phenomenon we are quite used to in mammals, although its basis in brain function is not understood, and one wonders why nature required a solution. Is learning not a process that goes on when an animal is awake and interacts with his environment? Perhaps in the echidna (and possibly in other monotremes with large prefrontal cortices ancestral to the echidna) this integration of new with older experience did take place during the waking state, and that is why it needed its outsized cortex. Nature's pressures for survival continued in the ever-changing environment. In the echidnalike monotremes even larger cortices may have been needed to provide additional perceptual and learning capacity. This was apparently not a productive direction for evolution to follow, for there is no evidence of a continued echidnalike line. Instead, in marsupial and placental mammals, nature hit upon a new solution to the problem of the integration of experience. The new solution, which allowed the same task to be performed with much less prefrontal cortex, was made possible by REM sleep. (The problem did not exist in the earlier reptilian species. The behavior of reptiles was largely reflexive, and this activity, as well as whatever small amounts of learning these animals acquired, was adequately handled by a small brain without a neocortex.)

Consider once again what we know of the prefrontal cortex. It is identified by its location at the frontal pole of the neocortex and its connections to a specific nucleus in the thalamus (the mediodorsal nucleus). It receives via input pathways all of the ongoing cognitive and emotional information available to the brain, and one of its major outputs is to the basal ganglia, a subcortical group of nuclei which is associated with action or movement. Recall Joaquim Fuster's view of the role of the frontal cortex in synthesizing behavior (page 59):

The most crucial constituents are the attentive acts that "palpate" the environment in search of significant clues, the intentional and elaborate movements, the continuous updating of relevant information, and the referring of that information to a cognitive scheme of the overall structure and its goal. The prefrontal cortex not only provides the substrate for these operations but imparts to them their active quality. In that active role . . . one may find some justification of the often espoused view of the prefrontal cortex as an agent—"the executive of the brain."

It appears then that the function of the prefrontal cortex is to formulate a strategy or plan for the future behavior of an animal so that it may take an appropriate action in a given situation. (This is clearly a different function from those performed by other parts of the neocortex, which detect and analyze incoming sensory stimuli and direct motor actions.)

We return to the echidna, and I hypothesize that the complex function of assimilating new information, associating it with memories of past experiences, and formulating a plan to govern new behavior adaptively during the waking state required a very large prefrontal cortex in this early mammal. (You may wish to refer back to Figure 9 on page 57.) It is clear that had the evolution of the brain proceeded along this line, higher mammals and man as we know them would never have been. For what occurred was that the new line of marsupial and placental mammals—lower-order animals like the echidna—had very small prefrontal cortices (the reason discussed below). As higher mammalian forms evolved, more and more cortical tissue was added (both prefrontal and other areas of neocortex) culminating in the brain of man, and this additional neural machinery provided many additional sensory, motor, and associative capabilities. Even with this evolutionary growth, man's prefrontal cortex did not grow to be as large a proportion of total cortex as it was in the echidna. Thus, should the organization of man's brain have been similar to the echidna's, he might have needed a wheelbarrow to carry it around. In short, man would not have evolved.

What was the scheme that nature hit upon in marsupial and placental mammals? I propose that it was, in computer terms, off-line processing. (Off-line processing is the acquisition of input information and its temporary storage in computer memory until a time when processing components are available.) The task of associating recent events to past memories and evolving a neural substrate to guide future behavior was accomplished when the animal was asleep. A small prefrontal cortex was sufficient because it did not have to work on this task of integration simultaneously with the processing of new information—it could perform its integrative function in a more leisurely manner during sleep. The new stage of sleep, REM sleep, was the crucial element (although not the whole story).

For support of this hypothesis we turn first to the hippocampus. Recall that the hippocampus is that central structure in the limbic system that is closely associated with memory. Our best understanding of its function is that it makes possible the registration in the brain of an event by drawing together all of the various sensory inputs that constitute the experience. We saw that for patients like H.M. without a hippocampus, memories of recent events are lost forever. We found that in the hippocampus, theta rhythm was generated in lower mammals during certain activities. We observed further that theta rhythm was in all likelihood the manifestation of a special form of neural processing of sensory information in lower mammals, originally evolved to coordinate all sensory input with cycles of sniffing in animals such as the rat, and then expanded to other activities in other species. These activities were important for the survival of each species. Taking the rat, cat, and rabbit for example, the activities during which theta rhythm occurred were exploration in all three species and, in addition, predatory behavior in the cat and escape from predation in the rabbit. Theta rhythm also occurred during one other state in all of the species —REM sleep, identified by its many physiological signs such as low amplitude, random cortical EEG, eye movements, loss of muscle tone in the limbs, and so on. I believe that the theta rhythm findings provide a clue to REM sleep information processing. Theta rhythm in lower mammals is a signature, a sign of the processing of sensory information. Its occurrence in REM sleep suggests that this sensory information is being processed once again, but this time in the sleeping state when there is no external sensory input.

The input information acquired earlier during activity is now taken from internal memory stores. And the fact that theta rhythm occurs only during certain species-specific waking activities provides another insight into REM sleep processing. In these lower mammals, not all experience is subject to reprocessing during REM sleep, with subsequent incorporation into a plan of behavior, but only experiences during certain activities of special importance to the species. As noted in Chapter 7, theta rhythm is found in the hippocampus of the echidna during burrowing behavior. There is no REM sleep in this animal, and no theta rhythm at all during sleep. Presumably, the large prefrontal cortex of the echidna is processing the information obtained during the waking state as it is acquired (in computer terms, the processing is on-line).

The theta rhythm data are suggestive of REM sleep processing of information. The work of my laboratory on neuronal gating in the hippocampus provides somewhat more definite evidence that such processing is indeed going on. I observed earlier that the means by which the hippocampus, in conjunction with the neocortex, performed its memory function are not yet understood. However, there was one definite finding. In functional terms, there was a switching of the path of information flow through the hippocampus during each of several behavioral states. Information was passed from the entorhinal cortex through the hippocampus to limbic system target structures that were different for each behavioral state. This rerouting of information is most readily interpreted as a change from one scheme (or, in computer terms, program) of information processing to another. And the behavioral states (in the rat) are those we have been discussing. In the rat's waking state, functional connectivity is different during exploration (with theta rhythm) than during the still-alert state (without theta rhythm). And in sleep, connectivity is different in slow-wave sleep from that in REM sleep. (We will return to the question of information processing in slow-wave sleep shortly.)

What kinds of experiences and memories are then processed in these lower mammals and used to build up a guide to future behavior? They would be the experiences and memories of exploration typified by the observation of Leyhausen in cats concerning their astounding ability, after one experience, to seek out many weeks later a particular place in a room or a piece of land in order to "look for more." Or experiences of predation in the cat—or escape from predators in the rabbit.

And now a very important point. After a time, certain of these strategies for behavior are not reversible or easily modified—presumably the critical period for connectivity in the prefrontal cortex has passed, and the strategy for behavior is largely set. An example may be Leyhausen's observation that kittens whose mothers do not bring live prey to them between their sixth and twentieth weeks, later do not kill or do it in a slow, laborious way.

There is other evidence for what occurs in lower mammals during REM sleep. There are Morrison's experiments, and those of Jouvet in which lesions in the brain stem of cats allowed the animals to move during REM sleep. These animals acted out attack and fear behavior—which in my view could represent activities being processed neurally during REM sleep as part of a laying down, integration, or rehearsal of predatory experience.

If REM sleep does indeed serve the function I suggest, then it is no wonder that it has been carried along in evolution without change from lower mammals to man—for it is a fundamental part of the functioning of the mammalian brain. And from this one can understand the origins of dreaming in man and what dreams represent. In man, dreams are a window on the neural process whereby, from early childhood on, strategies for behavior are being set down, modified, or consulted. (The experiences being evaluated and integrated in humans are no longer restricted to occurrences during particular activities, as they were in lower mammals, but now consist of all experience.) It is a matter of chance, not related to their function, that we are aware of dreams at all —and, of course, many people do not remember them. But dreams do reflect the processes we have been discussing. Further, when Freud dissected and analyzed dreams and from them constructed his concept of the unconscious, he was looking at this process.

I believe that the phylogenetically ancient mechanisms involving REM sleep, in which memories, associations, and strategies are formed and handled by the brain as a distinct category of information in the prefrontal cortex and associated structures, are in fact the Freudian unconscious.

Can this hypothesis explain the psychological phenomena Freud associated with the unconscious such as dream distortion, repression, and transference? And does it lead to an understanding of the meaning of dreams? Before attempting to answer these questions I want to consider some of the findings I have already related and some new data about human thought processes.

It would appear that our brains may be handling thoughts, below the level of our conscious awareness, all the time. For example, a common experience is to try to recall a recent incident, name, or place, find ourselves unable to come up with the desired memory, only to have it pop into our heads minutes or hours later. Clearly we have instituted a search through past memory, which has proved successful after some time. All the while we have been engaged in many waking activities, unaware of this mental process. We noted evidence for sleep processing in Chapter 2. As we drift off to sleep, we experience hypnogogic imagery. This is reported by subjects awakened during sleep-onset about as often as dreams are reported following REM sleep awakenings (on the order of seven out of ten times). The thoughts that occur at sleep onset are fragmented images or minidramas which seem totally different from our waking thoughts just before drifting off to sleep—they reveal an independent line of mental associations. Awakenings during non-REM sleep (slow-wave sleep in animals) also show the presence of fanciful imagery, and during REM sleep we know that we generate dreams. As I have stated, I believe information processing occurs during REM sleep, and the mental associations during other stages of sleep may or may not reflect similar processing.

In 1978, Howard Roffwarg and associates at the Montefiore Hospital and the Albert Einstein College of Medicine in New York performed an experiment which demonstrated something more—an orderly integration of experience into dreams of the sort I have postulated as a basic brain mechanism. The idea was ingenious. Starting from a given day, during every waking moment, nine subjects, college students, wore goggles which changed the color of everything they perceived. This was accomplished by lenses in the goggles that excluded blue and green wavelengths in the incoming light, making all visual imagery appear a shade of red. The subjects soon became accustomed to this altered coloration of their perceived world, which they called "goggle colored."

Starting with the wearing of the filtering lenses, Roffwarg and his colleagues were, in effect, tagging all visual input with a distinct color. They reasoned that whatever processing of experience was occurring during sleep-onset, non-REM sleep, or in dreams, they might be able to follow it via the color of the scenes their subjects reported upon awakening. The experiment was performed most carefully, utilizing a variety of controls, and the results did indeed reveal a pattern of processing in sleep.

The first part of the experiment was a period of seven to ten days in which the subjects became acclimated to the goggles without color-altering lenses. Then there was an altered-color period of five to eight days and finally a recovery period of three to four days with normal vision. For the entire course of the experiment, the subjects slept in the sleep laboratory, were monitored via EEG and eye movements to determine their stage of sleep, and awakened during periods of sleep-onset, non-REM, and REM sleep to report ongoing thoughts and dreams. When wakened from REM sleep the subjects reported dreaming in goggle color from the first night of wearing the goggles. Generally they had four REM periods each night. On the first night, the goggle-colored scenes appeared in the first dreams of the night but not in succeeding ones. The content of all dreams of the night were normal for the subject, unaffected by the wearing of the goggles, but in the first dream about half of the scenes appeared with exactly the same red coloration as was seen through the goggles by day.

On succeeding nights, the goggle color penetrated into later and later REM periods, so that by the fourth or fifth nights, dreams from all REM periods had scenes with goggle coloration (it appeared in 44 percent of the late night dreams by the fourth and fifth night of wearing the goggles). As red coloration entered the later dreams of the night, it also pervaded more and more of the earlier dreams, so that by the fourth and fifth night of wearing the filtering lenses, the color was in 83 percent of the first REM period dreams of these nights. Clearly Freud and others were correct in their observations that dreams contained day residues, information taken from the previous few days. But it was more than that—there was a systematic processing of that information, day by day, into later and later dreams of the night.

There was another interesting aspect of this processing—the intermixing of recent events with earlier memories. Whatever dream material was not colored was clearly derived from memories of earlier experience—and indeed, in some instances, events that had occurred before the experiment had even begun reappeared in dreams recolored red. There were also instances of both red-colored and normal-colored scenes appearing in the same dream. Thus, a room in which a subject stood was normal, but a scene he viewed through a window was tinted red. All of these results suggested some complicated interaction between recent experience and memory. The last experimental finding regarding REM sleep was that when the goggles were removed and the subjects experienced one day of normal vision, the goggle-induced red coloration virtually disappeared from all dreams.

Awakenings from sleep onset (which were carried out several times a night as the subjects returned to sleep after REM or non-REM awakenings) suggested that a different process was operative. Data here were not as complete as for REM sleep awakenings, but were sufficient to show that there was a strong goggle coloration in the images recalled. However, the coloration was not more prevalent early in the night, it was present in sleep-onset mentation throughout the night. Further, red imagery in sleep-onset reports did not drop off immediately after removing the goggles as did the red coloration in dreams, but persisted for three days. Finally, awakenings from non-REM sleep showed a weaker goggle effect than in dreams or sleep-onset images.

The Roffwarg experiment strongly suggests the existence of systematic but complex information processing during sleep. The findings of Larry Squire and associates cited in Chapter 1 raise the same issue of information processing occurring below the level of conscious awareness, but raises it in relation to memory.

Let us consider the consolidation of memory. It will be recalled that Squire found that during a slow process of memory consolidation extending over a period of some three years, memories requiring the hippocampus for their retrieval were converted to a form in which the hippocampus was no longer necessary. Thus, H.M. without a hippocampus could recall events prior to three years from the time of his operation (long-term memory), but not more recent memories. Presumably, during the three-year period, memories were repetitively reactivated, practiced, or rehearsed, the hippocampus acting with the neocortex and other parts of the brain in this process. Ultimately, memories so reactivated were presumably largely encoded in the neocortex. At any rate, the hippocampus was no longer crucial for their recall.

In what behavioral state does this reactivation take place? It may occur continuously in the waking state. Processes such as the subconscious search for a past name or event that we have mentioned may only be an inkling of a complex system of subconscious associations that are constantly being made in the waking state, and subconscious rehearsal of memories and associations while we are awake may account completely for the consolidation of memory that occurs in the neocortex over a period of several years. Or reactivation of associations may occur during any of the phases of sleep. Sleep-onset or non-REM mentation could be indicators of the flow of such associations. Alternatively, reactivation may occur during REM sleep. I have portrayed REM sleep as a process whereby the flow of recent events and past associations is tapped into and integrated into a guide for future behavior. This sampling of recent memory during REM sleep was not thought of as playing a part in the formation of long-term memory. It is possible, however, that all of long-term memory is consolidated via this process. (This is the most extreme assumption. I raise it as a possibility but do not propose it as part of my general hypothesis.) That is, only those memories that are reached in association with such integration are rehearsed (night after night) and finally stored permanently. This would be a vast amount of material (and thus could constitute all of long-term memory) for, as I mentioned, we assume that in man the REM sleep process no longer constructs a behavioral plan merely for species-specific behaviors such as exploration and predation, but includes all of man's experience.

Whatever the means by which the three-year period of consolidation takes place, I find in the work of sleep researchers support for the view that a brain system for information processing operates during sleep in man, and suggest that the hippocampal gating mechanism described in lower mammals may constitute, at least in part, its neural substrate.

If this system is truly what Freud observed and called the unconscious, we ask again, can it explain the characteristics of the unconscious that Freud identified such as the repression of dream content via dream distortion (symbolism, the need for representability, condensation, and displacement) and the unraveling of latent dream content by means of free association?

I believe that certain of these characteristics do follow as a natural consequence of my hypothesis. Thus, on the basis of my theory I would say that there is no dream censor distorting dream content to keep its meaning from conscious awareness. I see dream distortion not as a defense but as a reflection of the normal associative process by which experience is interpreted and integrated. Consider symbolism first. In the 1970s David Foulkes carried out a very thorough study of the dreams of children, aged three to fifteen, at the University of Wyoming. Each child was followed over a five-year period, spending nine nights over the course of each year in a sleep laboratory where he or she was monitored for sleep phases and awakened and questioned as to ongoing thoughts during sleep-onset, non-REM, and REM sleep. The purpose of the study was not psychoanalytical but was to capture children's dream content in an unbiased manner. Foulkes reported dreams and the thoughts reported on awakening from other sleep stages of a young girl Emily from the ages of eleven to fifteen. He noted that Emily was completely naive with respect to Freudian ideas. At age thirteen, Emily related the following episode to him on awakening from sleep-onset:

There was a bunch of people standing around and they were passing something around. I don't know what it was. I think it was something you wear, like a choker or bracelet or something. [Who were the people in this?] They were a bunch of girls my age. [Did you recognize them? Were they girls you really know?] No. [Where were they?] They were in a room and it was really small and they were all really close together. . . . I couldn't tell what kind of building it was. [Were you in it?] Yes . . . I was looking at the things that they were passing around. I was passing them around too. We were just sort of standing around. [Did you have any feelings?] No.

She had had a previous (REM awakening) dream a month earlier in which the same symbol, a choker, appeared. Emily had been riding in a car with a girlfriend and the friend's father. Emily's choker had been left in the road and, as her friend tried to retrieve it, the girl's father drove away, leaving her stranded there. In keeping with the purpose of the study, Foulkes did not question Emily on her ideas of the meaning of her dreams or its symbols, but he felt that the meaning of the symbol of the choker was clear enough to comment as follows:

> Both by the nature of the symbol itself and by the contexts in which it appears, it is tempting to view it as representing, denotatively, femaleness and, connotatively, the constraints Emily imagines anatomy to impose on her as yet vaguely apprehended destiny (the father wants nothing to do with it; it is part of a specifically constricting world that only girls can experience in common).

Let us postpone for a moment the question of why everything in a dream must appear in the form of a visual scene (the need for representability) and ask in what way a symbol could be chosen to represent the concept of shared femininity. Representing the vagina as itself would not suffice, for where would the sharing appear? Emily's associative process arrived at a natural solution—the choker had the basic shape of the female sexual organ, was associated with females by its use, and could be pictured in a dream as shared. Indeed one suspects from the work on feature detection in associative cortex we have discussed, that all objects with holes or cavities in them are in close associational proximity to one another in the neocortex, and an associational search from the image of a vagina for a symbol, which had the other necessary attributes in this content, would soon select an image like a choker.

(The idea that dream distortion is not a defense mechanism but an expressive means, and that symbols are chosen to represent a combined idea was first proposed by psychologist Calvin Hall of the University of California at Santa Cruz in the 1950s and 1960s. His conclusion was based on the recording and interpretation of thousands of dreams.)

This concept gains support from other observations. It is commonplace in dreams to have a boy or man use a gun in a context in which the meaning is unmistakably a penis. In other dreams a faucet may appear, clearly symbolizing a penis again (Hall gives an example in which a man turns a faucet on, coinciding with his having a nocturnal emission). In still other dreams a penis in an act of sexual intercourse is represented as just that, without symbolic modification. Presumably in the first dream the penis was being considered as an instrument of aggression; in the second there was perhaps a reference to urination, capable of being turned off; and in the third no other connotation was to be expressed other than what the dream said directly.

Freud's own example of symbolism, a hat with an upturned center portion and down-turned side sections appearing in the dream of the young married woman with agoraphobia, can be seen as the dual expression of her husband's genitals and being under the safe "cap" of marriage. Freud viewed the symbol as a disguise, the result of repression to prevent the young woman's sexual desires from breaking through into consciousness. According to the present interpretation, her unconscious mind, the functionally distinct brain system in which her experiences were integrated, was simply making the statement, without any disguise, that she was safe under the protection of marriage, which did also provide her with the benefit of her husband's genitals. The symbol of the hat that resembled genitals expressed the idea concisely. The fact that she resisted Freud's interpretation was indeed a matter of repression, the exclusion of an unpleasant thought from consciousness (which I will discuss below), but repression did not act on the dream itself—the dream was not distorted by a dream censor.

Another observation of psychoanalysis also argues against Freud's defense theory. It is a common occurrence in analysis for a symbol to appear over and over again in the dreams of a patient. The patient may have established its meaning beyond doubt by numerous instances of

free association or cases in which the meaning was directly apparent.
And yet the symbol continues to appear in the patient's dream expressing the same succinct message each time. There is no longer any disguise, and if disguise by a censor were the operative mechanism, one
would think that a new disguise would be adopted by the censor. The
fact that the symbol is repeated supports the view that it is merely a
visual means which, for that individual, most efficiently expresses a
particular unconscious concept.

Only a few words need be said about condensation in dreams. According to my hypothesis it would be the natural bringing together of
two or more entities that are closely associated with one another—a
concept not much different from Freud's, except that condensation
does not function as a disguise but as a means of representing an
unconscious idea. Thus in the Irma dream, Breuer and Freud's elder
half-brother were depicted as a composite figure. Freud's unconscious
was out to deprecate Breuer (Dr. M.). In real life, Freud was angry with
Breuer for opposing his theory of hysteria. Searching for a means of
denigration, association was made to Freud's elder brother, who had
also recently refused a proposition of Freud's and who possessed some
physical characteristics which, if grafted onto Dr. M., would carry out
the deprecatory task nicely—namely, a limp and a clean-shaven appearance. (This latter interpretation was provided by Erik Erikson who
pointed out that a clean-shaven face denoted a lack of manliness and
distinction in Freud's day. Breuer actually possessed a handsome
beard.)

Turning to the "need for representability," as a result of the fact that
dreams are always visual scenes, Freud observed that concepts which
are abstract must be translated into actions in order to be represented.
You will recall the word "superfluous" translated into a dream in which
there was a deluge of rain. Why are dreams always visual scenes or
sequences of them? An additional feature of dreams was noted by
psychiatrist Ernest Hartmann. The dreamer never feels that he can
exert free will in the dream. The script is written, and the dreamer just
acts in it. This may be a direct result of the phylogenetic origin of the
brain mechanism we have postulated as corresponding to the unconscious. Language and abstract concepts derived therefrom played no

part in the lower mammalian brain. The limbic-frontal cortical system governing interpretation of experience and planning operated solely on the basis of action, and this remains the case in man. Thus, abstract concepts arising with language, which are a large part of our experience, can only be integrated into our unconscious brain mechanism by translation into visual scenes and actions—giving rise to the witty, fascinating, and difficult-to-translate components of dreams Freud identified as transformed by the need for representability. An example, a dream of a young businessman in psychoanalysis, may serve to illustrate this process as well as the process of free association.

A woman friend of the young man named Bea Rich arrived in New York in a cab and passed through to another city, in the course of which the young man helped her with her luggage. The woman dropped a beach coat, which he considered a rag that he would ordinarily throw away, but he did not because it was a recent purchase with a price tag on it.

In the course of the analytic hour, a series of free associations, without any interpretation by the analyst, led to the conclusion that Bea Rich was "be rich," and the dream signified that getting rich had passed the young man by. He was, in fact, in the process of developing a new business that brought him the prospects of wealth, but the dream stated the unconscious conviction that this would not occur. The rag was the new business that he disliked and would throw away except for the money in it (the price tag). In free association to the cloth of which the beach coat was made, the fabric "jersey faille" came to mind. The business was in fact located in New Jersey, and although the word "faille" is ordinarily pronounced "file," the pronunciation "fail" was his first association.

What was new in the dream that was not known before? Not very much except that the young man believed consciously that his business stood every chance of being successful, and the dream expressed his unconscious statement of the opposite. Whatever deeper significance the dream may have had was not reached in the analytic hour.

As Freud did, let us look at the dream from the latent content upward. Let us say that the unconscious statement to be made was that the new business would fail and riches would pass the man by—and further that this statement had to be expressed via a sequence of events because the constraints placed on the brain mechanism corresponding to the unconscious as a result of its phylogenetic origin required it. Associational paths would be searched, the friend Bea Rich whom the young man had seen a few days previously would be encountered among the most recent experiences (day residue), and based on the double meaning of the name, this selection would be made. Similarly would "Jersey fail" cloth and a rag with a price tag be singled out, items of current experience which by dint of a pun or some other play on words could be utilized to express the message. These elements might indeed have been chosen because, as Freud would have it, they were overdetermined. Bea Rich might have had some further significance to the young man. In any case, the unconscious associational network utilized these symbols for a statement (the purpose of the statement will be addressed later). In this context we see that free association was truly a remarkable discovery of Freud's. When it is accomplished, it allows one to follow the associational paths of the search.

The last means of dream distortion that Freud identified was displacement. In particular he highlighted the displacement of emotion away from the manifest content of a dream (dream of the botanical monograph). Freud noted that displacement of this type was not common in dreams. I have no explanation for it in terms of my theory except that in the search for representability in the manifest dream, the emotional content may at times be sacrificed.

We come now to a most important characteristic of our unconscious brain system—its plasticity early in life and the fixing of its connections later. We have seen that the neurons of all of the neocortex, the prefrontal cortex included, are in an immature state at birth. Their dendrites and axons grow during the first few years of life, making interconnections which are affected by environmental stimuli during the critical period and then become largely permanent. The result, in the associative cortex which mediates language, is proficiency in the language to which a child has been exposed early on and a distinctive accent. However, in our system, the prefrontal cortex is being formed in response to experience, generating a many-faceted strategy or plan for living. Later this is hard to change, for patterns of reaction may be governed largely by fixed connections. The phenomenon of the critical period may be of benefit to lower mammals, giving them this ability to face life independently at an early stage of life, but it is not beneficial to man in whom all sorts of early misconceptions may become entrenched for an entire lifetime.

Going back a bit, I hypothesize that in the newborn infant, with the prefrontal cortex in an immature state, lower brain centers (such as the basal ganglia) govern activity. (This has been demonstrated by Patricia Goldman-Rakic of Yale University for certain behavioral tasks in monkeys.)* The neural process constituting REM sleep is likewise immature and nonfunctional. At birth there are sensitivities, clear differences among infants. And there are the sophisticated signs of emotionality—disdain, amusement, and such that Roffwarg and colleagues saw in the faces of infants during REM sleep. These may reflect inborn emotional components which will later react with experience in the formation of personality. By the age of two, the child is becoming aware of his or her own existence, and I postulate that impressions are rapidly being formed and integrated into the unconscious during off-line processing in REM sleep. This continues at a decelerating rate until the end of the critical period, an indefinite time perhaps as late as adolescence. REM sleep processing continues throughout life, but it is the earlier impressions, those acquired during the critical period, that are the basis for the interpretation of many later events. Above and beyond this there is normal learning, which grows throughout life.

What sorts of impressions are perceived and become part of the unconscious? The answer comes from psychoanalysis, and one may wish to treat it with caution in view of the problems of suggestibility in psychoanalysis we have discussed. However, little of what psychoanalysts have reported is to be discounted on the face of it, considering the brain mechanism I postulate whereby early misimpressions may be fixed and not available for correction later in life.

Certainly, an infant's separation from its parents even for a few weeks early in life may leave a lifelong fear of abandonment, an overdependence on a secure environment. Sexuality is a major source of disturbing ideas. The little boy does associate his penis with aggression.

A man may dream of pouring hot acid on the head of a father figure while a beautiful woman waits in the wings, and awake to a nocturnal emission. As already noted, dreams may show that a man believes unconsciously that he can gain phallic strength by incorporating his father's penis anally. Fantastic misconceptions of pregnancy appear in dreams as do many of the much-discussed dreams of killing siblings or parents. All of this affects normal personality and underlies neurosis when it occurs. Beyond this there is role playing—unconscious and at times consciously acted out trials of different strategies of behavior—a subject we will return to later.

With all of this said, we may now ask what is the meaning of dreams? I have mentioned several times that dreams of a given night appear frequently to deal with the same subject. Freud observed this, having access in all likelihood to less than the four or five dreams we each have every night, and sleep researchers have seen it when they obtain a report of every dream of the night. Rosalind Cartwright, professor of psychology at Rush Presbyterian St. Luke's Medical Center in Chicago, has monitored successive dreams of a night in volunteer medical students. The way the dreams of a medical student, Don, dealt with a single subject are what she found typical. They may give the reader a more concrete idea of the progression of a single theme.

The student's first dream was an elaborate story of being in a boardinghouse with large and small rooms. Oddly, one could see from one room to the other through gratings. A tenant had been killed by another tenant, and the man who did it was organizing an effort to get rid of the body. Rolls of paper, held together by a sticky, gelatinlike glue, were being used to cover the corpse. Helping the killer was his girlfriend, a not very pretty girl with long black hair.

The subject had had two experiences on the day before the night spent in the laboratory, and Cartwright found both incorporated into the first dream. The first was that, as a medical student, he had dissected his first cadaver; this was an adult male, whose body was delivered wrapped in brown paper. The second was the preparatory activity the student had experienced in the sleep laboratory itself. He saw sheaves of paper being loaded into the EEG machine, and sticky, gelatinlike collodion was used to fix recording electrodes to his scalp. Also, the sleep laboratory did have both large and small rooms from which one could observe the goings on in adjacent areas. Cartwright could identify the killer as the laboratory assistant who applied the collodion and loaded the paper and the girlfriend as herself. This first dream then contained the day residue. It also served as an example of the penetration of events of the day into the first REM dream of the night as was seen in the red-goggles experiment. In later questioning, Cartwright determined the further fact that the subject had just moved into a boardinghouse, his first time of living away from home. It was full of homosexuals, and he wanted to move out but could not for practical reasons.

The second dream found the student on the South Side of Chicago in a tough black neighborhood. In real life, his father used to have a drugstore in the area. He was with a friend, and they were being followed by two junkies, about forty or fifty years old, who were getting belligerent. They demanded a dime from the student's friend and then a dollar. When this was not forthcoming, they grew more threatening. The student went into a phone booth and tried to call his father, but could not make himself understood to the operator. When he was awakened, the subject remembered feeling fear.

Cartwright ascertained that an incident of this kind had in fact occurred some time in the past. The student had been followed into a drugstore in that neighborhood. The pharmacist had phoned the police, who drove the student home. Cartwright noted a theme in the dreams thus far—entrapment in close quarters, menaced by sinister people.

The third dream was a classic Freudian wish fulfillment. The student found himself in an expensive outdoor café in Paris amidst the upper strata of society, calmly sipping Bordeaux. The wish clearly was for a complete escape from his problems.

In the fourth dream, the student returned to his concerns, which took a turn toward sexuality. He dreamed that he was giving riding lessons to a pretty girl. He and a friend also picked up two other girls. When the girl he was teaching to ride got on her horse, she decided that it was easiest to make it go faster by jamming a fountain pen into its rump, and this maneuver worked.

Cartwright saw the dream as a tentative turn toward heterosexuality, which received a rebuff in a masculine-acting girl. She began to discern that the whole dream series was dealing with the issue of the student's unconscious ideas about sexuality.

The fifth and last dream of the night had the student driving a car to a concert with a girl he didn't like very much but whom he took because she had a car. Plans were changed, and they decided to see a movie. To quote an excerpt from this dream:

> We started back and we were going to see a movie. At the S-turn on the Outer Drive, we got into some sort of an accident and held up traffic there. This girl I had taken in her car—which is, as I remember, the reason that I took her to the concert was that she had a car—she is some girl in my class here in school. I don't like her very much at all. She is not very pretty and so she compensates by not being very nice also. One of the reasons I had the accident on the S-curve is that it was packed with 150-story buildings on both sides of the street. They had built these towering, towering skyscrapers and I had never seen these before and I was so shook by all these that I was looking at the skyscrapers and I went straight instead of turning and just hit a wall.

Cartwright saw this dream as saying that the student found going with girls unsatisfactory, experienced being surrounded by large phallic figures and lost control although he tried to "go straight."

Cartwright did not question her subject closely on the meaning of his dreams—her research concerned the content of a dream series. The student did volunteer the information that he had his own car and did not need the girl's. A psychoanalyst listening to these dreams would not be surprised if this young man, as predicted by the unconscious material, ended up married to a dominating female as an escape from homosexuality.

What does this series tell us about the meaning of dreams? It seems that a single important problem is being considered. New experiences are being interpreted in the light of that problem. The dreams are by no means wish-fulfilling except for one which is a classic example.

Cartwright has found that a wish-fulfilling dream is frequently embedded in a series of dreams that are not.

Pursuing the question of the meaning of dreams, let us now turn, to Freud's Irma dream. But first, a short dream which I believe is similar in theme.

The dream was that of a middle-aged actor whose five-year psychoanalysis had been completed some time before the dream occurred. It pictured a storm at sea. There was a lost duckling, which seemed to the actor to be himself, in distress in the impossible seas. A torpedo boat with a captain was looking for the duckling, which now turned into a poor dog. The captain had a turned collar like a priest. The dreamer had the conviction that the poor dog would be saved.

Upon a little reflection, the dreamer was able to come up with what he considered to be the meaning of the dream. Having been quite successful in his career, he was now in financial trouble—drowning in financial seas. The duckling was a clear reference to an infant in an Anthony Trollope novel that his wife was reading and had discussed with him. In the novel, the infant was fought for by a father, separated from his wife, the infant's mother. The mother constantly referred to her baby, a boy, as her little duckling. The actor not only saw himself as a helpless infant but as a "poor dog." The turned collar identified the torpedo boat captain as a priest—that is, a "father." And the message of the dream was the unconscious wish or perhaps conviction that the actor's father would rescue him from his current dilemma.

Now the man in this case was actually facing his financial problem resolutely. Nowhere in his conscious thinking was there any thought of himself as a helpless child. And indeed his father would be the last one he could turn to for help. For now retired, his father had been a failure in his small business and was being partially supported by the actor. But the actor's unconscious mind ignored all of this and looked back to a childhood expectation of rescue. And so the meaning of the dream was that the father would help, and I believe Freud was expressing a similar sentiment in his Irma dream.

You will recall Freud's analysis of his Irma dream. Freud's conclusion was that the dream represented a wish fulfillment. Blame for Irma's condition (her infection in the dream but her incompletely cured hysteria in real life) was Otto's, not his. In the article discussing the un-published Freud-Fliess correspondence, which disclosed the traumatic operation Fliess performed on Emma's (Irma's) nose, Max Schur sug-gested that the real work of the dream was to remove blame of the mishap from Fliess and place it on Otto, in addition to removing blame from Freud for his incomplete cure of her hysteria:

> But it was not only his own exculpation that he achieved, it was the need to exculpate Fliess from responsibility for Emma's nearly fatal complications that was probably the strongest (immediate) motive for the constellation of his dream.

Schur surmised that Freud's inability to note the similarity of the con-tent of the dream to the actual event of Fliess's operation on Emma several months earlier was due to repression. Freud needed Fliess's friendship (Schur termed it a deeper attachment, a transference) and therefore would not allow the similarity to enter his conscious thoughts. (The exclusion of thoughts from the conscious mind via the mechanism of repression does clearly exist and will be discussed shortly. This is not the same as repression acting to disguise dream content, which Freud assumed to be a basic mechanism of dream formation and which I postulate is not operative in the formation of dreams.)

The similarity of the incidents in the Irma dream to Emma's actual operation were noted by Schur and pointed out in even greater detail by psychoanalysts Ramon Greenberg and Chester Pearlman in an arti-cle in 1978. (These authors provided an alternate interpretation of Freud's dream as an unconscious attempt at adaptation—that is the dream helped Freud to defend against emotion arising from the inci-dent, to adapt to the situation of resenting Fliess's action but needing him.) Indeed the Irma dream portrays Emma's operation with com-plete fidelity—Freud's alarm at her condition, the white patch in the region of the turbinal bones (the gauze left by Fliess in his operation of the turbinate bone and sinus), the calling in of Leopold in the dream, a careful more deliberate physician after Otto had caused the trouble (the cautious consultant Dr. R. called in to repair Fliess's damage in the actual incident). There is little doubt that Freud was re-creating the incident in his dream, and I suggest that the formulation and the meaning of the dream was the following:

In real life, Otto came to see Freud on the day of the dream bringing him news of Emma's remaining hysterical symptoms and a gift of liqueur, smelling like fusel oil. This was the day residue and the reason that Otto appeared in the dream. The Irma dream was probably one of a series that night dealing with the adequacy of his psychoanalytic theories and his treatment of Emma. Smelling the spoiled liqueur was perhaps a key stimulus—it was promptly associated with the foul-smelling iodoform pack Dr. R. had removed from Emma's nose. The dream therefore stated flatly that Fliess had made the dirty injection—Freud's unconscious was in effect saying, "Thank you, Fliess, for making me a gift of a foul-smelling iodoform pack and almost killing my patient." The dream called attention to Fliess in the strongest possible fashion— the word "trimethylamin" was spelled out in heavy type—but rather than see the connection to Fliess's blunder, Freud chose to associate this word with the thought that Fliess was a friend whose "sympathy I remember with satisfaction whenever I feel isolated in my opinion." (I have pointed out that Freud's thoughts about Fliess's blunder may have been repressed as Schur suggested or, conceivably, they were deliberately not mentioned though they were remembered, because Freud felt they were not relevant to the meaning of the dream. In neither case did Freud admit to himself his anger at Fliess nor see that the dream expressed it.)

And the rest of the dream was Freud's call for help, a reliance on Breuer to rescue him. Breuer had befriended Freud in medical school and supported him both personally and financially. Freud's entire career was launched by Breuer's cathartic method. And this was exactly what Freud was depending on to pull him out in the case of Emma. Dr. M.'s comment that "dysentery will follow, and the poison will be eliminated" was not a foolish remark but Freud's hope and wish that Breuer's cathartic method which he was using to treat Emma (named indeed in analogy with catharsis of the digestive tract) would cure his patient. In all, the dream did not remove blame from anyone, neither Freud nor Fliess. Its entire statement was this: Fliess is responsible for putting my patient Emma in a bad way, but Breuer's cathartic method will save her.*

If one wants to speculate further (and this is indeed far-reaching speculation) one can illustrate another one of Freud's conclusions, namely that unconscious motivation can underlie many of our individual actions. Freud was in close correspondence with Fliess on every aspect of *The Interpretation of Dreams* as he wrote it. Why of all dreams did he pick the Irma dream as his specimen dream and bring it so closely to Fliess's attention? The action may have been guided unconsciously. The dream, at least the portion concerning Irma's infection, was really quite obvious. Freud may have unconsciously wanted to get the message across to Fliess, although the message was repressed and kept from his conscious awareness.

Before attempting to formulate a final answer to the question of the meaning of dreams, let us look at one more aspect of dreaming, the dreams that occur in psychoanalysis under the influence of transference. Transference is a most unusual phenomenon. The mere entry into psychoanalysis frequently produces intense unconscious reactions. Within the first few sessions of a psychoanalysis that is taking hold, the subject may dream of violently attacking or being attacked by the analyst. Something in the patient's knowing that he will soon be revealing his deepest feelings and will be vulnerable to deep psychological hurt provokes this reaction. The patient also knows he will be dependent on the analyst and thus turns the attention of the unconscious back to the events of early childhood. Dreams then tend to center on early experiences and impressions. And it is here that dreams reveal the bizarre and perverse ideas of sexuality, sibling rivalry, and the like. In an analysis that is progressing, dreams at this level predominate, going over such material again and again and revealing different attitudes of the dreamer to the same concerns. For example, Oedipal dreams may either reflect attacking a father or being attacked by him—and neither unconscious idea is necessarily based on the real relationship that existed between the father and young son.

What then is the meaning of dreams? On the basis of our theoretical formulation, we would not expect a simple answer. Dreams may be expected to have all of the variability and scope of conscious thinking and, in addition, may be expected to reflect many unconscious associations and memories. Nonetheless we can pick out certain characteristics of dreams. Dreams tell things as they are in the unconscious mind (that is, as they are registered in the functional subsystem of the brain we have discussed). For example, Freud's Irma dream expressed his knowledge of Fliess's blunder and his hope for the cathartic method. The young businessman's dream expressed the unconscious conviction that riches had passed him by, although consciously he believed in his success. In psychoanalysis or when life's concerns bring them up, dreams may reflect ideas of sexuality, power, or abandonment. There are also wishes as Freud proposed, similar to conscious thoughts in which we say, "If only this were so."

From his clinical experience, Jung derived a description which corresponds to what I propose here:

> The dream gives a true picture of the subjective state while the conscious mind denies that this state exists or recognizes it only grudgingly . . . when we listen to the dictates of the conscious mind we are always in doubt . . . The dream comes in as the expression of an involuntary psychic process not controlled by the conscious outlook. . . . It represents the subjective state as it really is.

Indeed, if one had access to and could analyze one's dreams every night, one could find a continuous series of thoughts on the most important aspects of one's life, free of rationalization and often startling in what they reveal about motivation.

I would venture to carry the analysis of dreams one step further. The scope of the unconscious ideas that occur in an individual's dreams appear to be so broad-ranging—sexual orientation and desires, self-image, insecurities as well as secure areas and grandiose ideas, jealousy and love, strategies for coping with the real world—and so interrelated in their viewpoint that I suggest they may best be described as constituting a personality: the *unconscious personality* of the dreamer.

I suggest then that dreams are the statements, wishes, hopes, and fears of the unconscious personality. Their night-to-night content—

that is, what captures the interest of our unconscious personality—is to some extent dependent on life's events. Psychoanalysis has a special influence; in psychoanalysis, the Oedipal and other familial conflicts in one's life frequently take over. Dream content may be violent. It is as if a small demon were in the unconscious ready to do battle. There are other ideas held by the unconscious personality that are startling and repugnant to one's conscious self. Freud's jealousy of his son and wishing him dead is an example. Life's real circumstances are often the subjects of concern—the actor's worry about his finances, Freud's doubts about his abilities as a physician in treating Irma, the fears of Rosalind Cartwright's student Don about his potential homosexuality are instances. But at times real problems of the most urgent nature are ignored. A patient may be diagnosed as having a life-threatening disease resulting in a deep state of anxiety or depression. Yet his or her dreams may go blithely on for weeks dealing with other matters. The situation may then be acknowledged in a dream that is realistic or in a wish-fulfilling dream of a cure. Dreams may also recount conscious decisions, complete with the conscious reasoning by which they were made.

The unconscious personality looks at the world in its own way, according to its own strategy for survival. What determines dream content of a given night is a matter for future investigation. But one feature of dreams and the unconscious personality is outstanding: The motivations underlying and guiding behavior in many of the important areas of our lives are to be found there.

This last concept, the unconscious personality, requires further psychoanalytic data for its evaluation. I discuss it further in the final chapter of this book.

Before concluding my theory of the biological basis of the unconscious, I wish to consider one further source of data. This is the study of children's dreams carried out by David Foulkes and referred to earlier in this chapter. As the reader will recall, children ranging from the ages of three to fifteen were monitored in the sleep laboratory for nine nights during the year where they were awakened from sleep-onset, non-REM, or REM sleep and asked to tell their thoughts. The study was designed in such a way that a given child could be followed for several years (either in a lower or upper age group) so as to observe the development of dreams in individual children rather than merely to obtain a sampling from many children of each age. Foulkes found that three- to five-year-olds dreamed straightforward stories of their simple wants and pleasures such as sleeping and eating. There was little action and no strong emotions. The characters in their dreams were themselves, members of their families, and familiar animals (perhaps representing themselves). By the age of seven, there were fewer themes relating to sleep and fatigue and more social interactions, about one fourth of which involved aggressive encounters. Dream symbolism started to appear. Dreams were still quite unlike adult dreams; they were not complex narratives but short episodes—playing with a friend or running a race.

In the seven- to nine-year-olds' dreams there were fewer animals and more humans, including strangers. Aggressive social encounters continued, and the children at this age reported their first experiences of feelings within dreams (as opposed to their feelings about dreams when awakened, which were always present). From the ages of nine through thirteen, the preadolescent years, dreams began to take on the fantasy characteristics of adult dreams. In content, the outside world was explored more widely. The first reports of fear appeared in dreams, and symbolism became prominent—Emily's dreams about her choker, related earlier, occurred at the age of thirteen. Foulkes's final sample dreams were from the age range of thirteen to fifteen. There were no striking changes in this adolescent period—symbolism reached an adult stage of development.

Foulkes concluded that children's dreams went along with the concerns of the children's lives and were also limited by and reflected their cognitive capability of representing the outside world at any given age. He observed further that symbols did not arise as dream distortions but as "new toys that children's cognitive development gives them a chance to play with"—a concept we put forth earlier in this chapter. None of this was especially surprising. What was surprising however, was an almost complete lack of the bizarre anatomical, sexual, and aggressive material (addressed to siblings and parents) which is so prominent in adult dreams and presumably is derived from childhood.

In summarizing his study, Foulkes commented that although there may indeed be an infantile and childhood unconscious, "our data do refute the hypothesis that dreaming is the 'royal road' to the discovery of this [unconscious] world and that dreaming is the quintessential product of this [unconscious] world."

There are several possible explanations for the contradiction between Foulkes's findings and all that has gone before. The most obvious is that, under the conditions of his experiment, he did not get the dreams that contain this material. He sampled dreams only nine nights in the year and under special circumstances—those of the laboratory where special psychological conditions prevail. It has been noted by dream researchers that laboratory dreams lack much of the sexual content and aggressive interactions that are present in dreams recorded the morning after a night's sleep at home. Reinforcing this possibility is the widespread experience of parents and child psychiatrists of the occurrence of frightening dreams and nightmares in children (Foulkes did not record a single nightmare).* Foulkes was of course aware of this effect but believed that it did not substantially affect his results. Further research should be able to resolve this issue, but Foulkes's findings bring to mind another possible explanation which would, in any case, deserve consideration.

In my theory of the biological origin of dreaming, dreams on a given night reflect a particular concern of the dreamer and the calling up of material relevant to this concern from the unconscious—impressions and experience integrated over time from childhood on. These current concerns in children are what Foulkes observed. In adult dreams, they are exemplified by Freud's Irma dream, the young businessman's "Bea Rich" dream, and the actor's dream in which his father will save him from drowning. The powerful, bizarre dream content we have encountered in our discussions has been associated with a few specific aspects of life, primarily sexuality and aggression. Taking sexuality as an example, it is not until preadolescence or adolescence that this activity becomes a concern of life. Therefore, in the light of my theory, it would not be surprising if it were found that sexuality played a minor role in children's dreams. That is not to say that all of the frequently misconceived infantile and childhood impressions of sex are not registered in memory. I would postulate that they are, along with such experiences as early feelings of pleasure in childhood masturbation. However, only in adolescent or adult years when sex does become a major preoccupation, and the associative networks are called upon to govern attitudes and behavior in this area, would these early impressions surface. Thus, this material would appear in adult dreams, which deal with sexuality, and not in children's dreams, which do not. This hypothesis would also explain the odd blend of relatively sophisticated symbolism and information about sex (acquired in later childhood or adolescence) with infantile ideas about anatomy and the like. An example might be the construction of the Oedipal fantasy partly from early childhood impressions of the sexual act and the desire of the young boy for the exclusive love and attention of the mother and partly from the later understanding of sexual possession. To summarize this view, dreams can indeed be considered the royal road to the unconscious, but there are several roads going to different places in the unconscious at different ages.

I have now completed my theory of the unconscious. In lower mammals it was the complete neural system needed to learn from experience, build up a plan for purposeful behavior, and survive. I hypothesize that in the course of evolution a new neural mechanism was added —that responsible for consciousness of oneself and the world. This is an assumption in two respects. It is evident that humans have such consciousness but a case can be made (and has been by Donald Griffin, professor of animal behavior at the Rockefeller University) that animals possess this capability also but are hampered in communicating it by their lack of language. Secondly, there are a number of neuroscientists who believe that consciousness is not generated in the neural networks of the brain but is derived from a nonphysical, spiritual source. A leading proponent of the spiritual view is Sir John Eccles, Nobel prizewinner for his work in the neurophysiology of the spinal cord. The opposite argument, that consciousness is based in the brain, is held by many neuroscientists and has been stated by Roger Sperry, who won the Nobel prize for his work in split-brain patients.* Freud of course held the same view. Since there is virtually no evidence either way, one's opinion on this subject is a matter of faith. My own belief is that consciousness, like the unconscious, is generated in the brain.

Regardless of its source, man does have consciousness, and it is the interplay of the conscious with the unconscious that we consider now. I have postulated that the neural system constituting the unconscious was in place before consciousness in man arose. There was apparently no functional necessity for our conscious mind to be aware of thought processes going on in the phylogenetically earlier unconscious subsystem of the brain. Neither was there an absolute bar to it, and thus dreams may be remembered or not. I have also described a third functional brain entity, which we may call the preconscious, the thought processes probably going on constantly beneath the level of conscious awareness. A process such as the instituting of an associational search is in this category. Such processes are not conscious, but neither are they part of the unconscious, the neural system responsible for the formulation of a behavioral strategy. They appear to be closely allied with consciousness. The associational search, for example, is begun by a conscious mental act. This third functional brain entity, consisting of those processes which are neither conscious nor part of the unconscious, are close enough to what Freud called the preconscious to use his terminology. The term "subconscious" could also be used. If the three-year process that consolidates memory takes place during the waking state, as does the associative search, then it would be considered a preconscious (or subconscious) process, since it is not consciously perceived and not part of the mechanism corresponding to the unconscious I have described.

It is in the interaction of conscious and preconscious that we find some of the mechanisms that Freud and others observed. Repression is one of them. It is clearly operative in keeping painful thoughts from consciousness. If one accepts Schur's explanation that Freud refused to admit Fliess's treatment of Emma to his conscious mind, then this is a prime example of repression. Amnesia for intense trauma such as war experiences is another. Displacement of an emotion from one person to another is a second mechanism that we can ascribe to preconscious-conscious interaction, when the emotion arises from a realistically hurtful or threatening experience. The man who is angry at a superior at work and then comes home to vent his anger at the members of his family using flimsy excuses is an instance. (There may, in addition, be

unconscious involvement. The man's anger may not be justified realistically but may be derived from a transference—for example, unconscious association of his superior with an early figure in his life like his
father.)*

There is in fact one neuropsychological study that does bear on the
question of consciousness and on repression in particular. A series of
experiments was performed by Benjamin Libet and associates at Mt.
Zion Hospital in San Francisco during the 1960s and 1970s on patients
being treated for Parkinson's disease or for chronic intractable pain. By
applying an electrical stimulus to the skin of one hand, which the
patient could feel and report, and applying a second stimulus directly to
the neocortical area governing skin sensation, which the patient felt as
a somewhat different tingling sensation in the skin of the same hand,
Libet and his colleagues were able to demonstrate that in order for a
sensation to become conscious, processing was required somewhere in
the brain and that this processing took about one half second. Ordinarily this would result in a bizarre condition; our skin would be
touched, and we would not feel it for one half second. However, to
maintain the normal simultaneity we sense between the touching of
the skin and the subjective feeling that it is being touched, Libet found
that the brain registered the subjective event as occurring one half
second earlier than when the processing of the subjective sensation was
completed. That is, the brain mechanism producing conscious sensation corrected for its own processing time in order to attain subjective
simultaneity.

Libet's experiments are described in more detail in Notes and References.* These experiments are unique and important since they point
to consciousness as the result of a distinct neural process. Although the
process is unknown, the one-half second required for a sensation to
become conscious appears to provide a neuropsychological basis for
repression in that there is time for other associative processes in the
functional entity we call preconscious to analyze events, thoughts, and
memories and repress them if their content is too painful.

We have arrived at three functional brain entities: the unconscious, a
particular body of information built up and processed in the limbic-
prefrontal system; the conscious, all of our immediate knowledge of

ourselves and the world; and the preconscious, complex associations perhaps occurring all of the time, without our awareness. What is their interaction? Besides the few findings we have been able to present, it is not understood. But their interaction is responsible for normal personality development, abnormal mental states—such as neurosis and psychosis, and phenomena such as multiple personality and hypnosis.* To close this chapter I will discuss these matters, not to present any real hypothesis but in the attempt to encompass the whole issue in some framework, however inadequate. Some of the hints I will use are observations I have already related and a few new findings.

Let us consider neurosis first. It seems quite apparent that the symptoms of classic neuroses express stubbornly fixed unconscious thoughts of an irrational and self-destructive nature. How else can one explain a hand-washing compulsion in which the patient reveals the idea that he must wash constantly or he will poison someone with dirty hands? In what other way can one understand a case of anorexia nervosa (a syndrome of indefinite classification) in which a young woman, emaciated by self-starvation, looks in a mirror and finds herself fat. And these ideas are influenced by the general societal environment. Hysteria in Charcot's time was more prevalent among country girls than among the more sophisticated girls of the city—and it is almost gone now.* Anorexia nervosa is apparently increasing in this day of emphasis on body image. Do these unconsciously mediated conditions have a physical basis? Yes—it all has a physical basis if unconscious ideas are processed and fixed in the brain as I have described. And some neuroses are beginning to yield to psychoactive drugs. Why is it that some people become neurotic and others not, while dealing with the same type of unconscious material? Perhaps it is an inborn tendency as Jung and Freud suggested—a tendency in which heredity biases the brain in some very subtle way. And the influence of individual experience on this tendency to neurosis (as distinct from its influence on the content of neurotic ideas) cannot be excluded, for emotions resulting from experience alter brain neurotransmitters and hormones which act physically on the brain.

What about those rare but fascinating cases of multiple personality? The psychoanalyst Lawrence Kubie has said that we will not understand the mind until we understand multiple personality. Psychoanalysis does give a clue. Patients in long-term analyses do reveal that their unconscious minds weigh alternate attitudes and strategies. A heterosexual may dream of homosexual solutions for his Oedipal conflicts and may feel and act out these strategies for a few days—not sexually but perhaps in his relations with men around him. Thus the normal mind may be constituted so as to consider, in early years, alternate strategies of behavior, alternate personalities. However, one personality emerges as the final one, the others to be discarded as a guide to behavior and glimpsed only occasionally in psychoanalysis. In multiple personalities, these alternate strategies with concurrent personality characteristics may rise to consciousness and periodically take over from one another. A precipitating factor may be overwhelming stress that the main personality cannot handle, especially in childhood.

It is interesting that multiple personalities can be called out and treated best by hypnosis. Kubie was very interested in hypnosis. A series of experiments led him to the conclusion that the essential element for inducing hypnosis was the restriction of sensory input to a minimum— a single sensory modality. Kubie hypnotized subjects merely by having them rest quietly and listen to the sounds of their own breathing transmitted through earphones. While in this hypnotic state, a suggestion transmitted through the earphones by an observer was adopted by the subject as part of his own thoughts. According to Kubie, this was the basis for hypnotic suggestion.

In addition to the tie between hypnosis and multiple personality mentioned above, other possible connections have been reported. Ernest Hilgard, professor of psychology at Stanford University, has induced by hypnosis multiple conscious entities in normal subjects, one observing the other. Kubie cites a case of a soldier who was hypnotized and told to return to a series of earlier stages in his own life. At each of these artificial earlier ages, the subject was put through a series of psychological and intelligence tests, and performed as though he actually was the hypnotically imposed age. The findings are suggestive—it appears that subpersonalities can be organized—but the process remains among the most mysterious of the mental phenomena.

It is in the mood disorders, depression and manic-depressive psychosis, as well as in schizophrenia that the strongest links to physical brain function have been found. As I noted in an earlier chapter, patients suffering from depression respond favorably to the drugs that act on the neurotransmitters norepinephrine and serotonin. Ordinarily these neurotransmitters are believed to fine-tune neural systems of the brain for a special situation. We have seen that norepinephrine may adjust function in the hippocampus, neocortex, and other brain areas to prepare the brain to respond to an alerting stimulus in the environment (the conditions calling forth serotonin modulation are unknown). In my own laboratory my colleagues and I have found that norepinephrine modulates neuronal gating in the hippocampus. These modulators, performing their tuning function in the normal brain, are in a position to produce serious abnormalities when their level is too low or too high— and this may occur in depression.

Manic-depressive psychosis—a different psychiatric condition from depression—responds to another chemical substance, lithium. The way lithium acts on the brain is unknown.

Schizophrenia, the last disease to be considered (in fact a group of related diseases), is in a class by itself. It is a disintegration of personality. From his vantage point at the Burghölzli, Bleuler described it as follows:

> In every case we are confronted with a more or less clear-cut splitting of the psychic functions. If the disease is marked, the personality loses its unity; at different times different psychic complexes seem to represent the personality. Integration of different complexes and strivings appears insufficient or even lacking. The psychic complexes do not combine in a conglomeration of strivings with a unified resultant as they do in a healthy person; rather, one set of complexes dominates the personality for a time, while other groups of ideas or drives are "split off" and seem either partly or completely impotent. Often ideas are only partially worked out, and fragments of ideas are connected in an illogical way to constitute a new idea. Concepts lose their completeness, seem to dispense with one or more of their essential components;

indeed, in many cases they are only represented by a few truncated notions.

Jung's description was:

The real trouble begins with the disintegration of the personality and the divestment of the ego-complex of its habitual supremacy . . . not even multiple personality, or certain religious or "mystical" phenomena, can be compared to what happens in schizophrenia. . . . It is as if the very foundations of the psyche were giving way. . . .

As a result of a determined research effort in recent years, a few scientific findings related to schizophrenia have emerged. The disease appears to be linked to dopamine (the third neurotransmitter of the monoamine class besides norepinephrine and serotonin) since drugs that are effective in ameliorating the symptoms of schizophrenia block the action of dopamine in the brain, and drugs that increase dopamine function exacerbate the symptoms. (There may also be a link to norepinephrine.) If a dopamine malfunction is at least in part the cause of schizophrenia, the propensity for malfunction may be inherited, for careful studies have suggested some degree of genetic transmission in schizophrenia. In view of what we have seen so far about the site of the neural networks underlying personality, one might begin to look for an abnormality in the prefrontal cortex of schizophrenics. One study has indicated such an abnormality.

The study was performed by David Ingvar at the University Hospital, University of Lund, in Sweden. The rate of blood flow in various regions of the neocortex was measured by having patients inhale a radioactive gas, which could be followed in the blood as it flowed through the brain by radiosensitive counters placed around the head. Regional blood flow is an indicator of the degree of neuronal activity in a region—a high rate of blood flow indicates active neurons and vice versa. Ingvar measured blood flow in normal subjects lying quietly with minimal external stimulation and showed blood flow in the frontal region of the neocortex to be 20 percent to 40 percent higher than in other regions. In Ingvar's words:

> The high frontal activity suggests that in the resting conscious state—unaccompanied by movements, speech or behavioral reactions—the brain is active with an anticipating stimulation of behavior.

This finding is obviously consistent with the view of frontal cortical function we have been hypothesizing. In schizophrenic patients, Ingvar found low cerebral blood flow in frontal regions and high flow in certain other parts of the neocortex. The frontal cortex was far less active.

Schizophrenia may not only be (or may not be at all) a prefrontal cortical malfunction. There is little information available. Malfunction at some critical link of the limbic system may be a causative factor. How may dopamine (or norepinephrine) be involved? Again these neurotransmitters are performing a normal function at most stages of this limbic system. Abnormal release of the transmitters at any point could create havoc. And there is another possibility. There are high levels of dopamine and norepinephrine in the frontal cortex. In the visual cortex, it has been found by John Pettigrew and Takaji Kasamatsu at the California Institute of Technology that norepinephrine may serve a double function. We have already indicated that norepinephrine may tune the visual system so as to be more efficient in processing incoming visual information during a state of alertness. Experiments by Pettigrew and Kasamatsu have suggested that norepinephrine may act in young animals, during the critical period, to help establish the connections within the visual cortex that are being made on the basis of visual experience. Without norepinephrine the connections do not become set. The opposite is also true. In an adult cat, with visual connections presumably fully set for life, the addition by external means of extra norepinephrine loosens the connections—replasticizes them. One could imagine that excess dopamine or norepinephrine in the prefrontal cortex of schizophrenics, introduced by abnormal neurotransmitter released within the brain, might have a similar effect of replasticizing the prefrontal circuits mediating personality. All of this is conjecture of course. The answer will come from experiments.

With this description of mental disease, I have completed the presentation of my theory and turn to my final chapter—a discussion of its experimental evaluation and its implications.

Ten

EPILOGUE

Dreams are the window of the unconscious. Freud made that point clear. Why do human beings dream? A complex process such as dreaming during REM sleep does not spring full blown into a species without an evolutionary history, and indeed we have that history in the development of REM sleep from the earliest marsupial and placental mammals to man. What is the function of REM sleep in animals? I have found it to be a basic physiological mechanism by which strategies of behavior based on an animal's experience are gradually constructed—a mechanism important for survival. The function of human dreaming cannot be far removed. That again is the way of evolution. And so I believe that the content of dreams reflects a strategy for behavior in man. But behavioral strategies are set early in an animal's life because of the critical period. And similarly in humans it is set in early childhood by our critical period. The result is the unconscious, a panoply of conceptions and misconceptions, gathered in the earliest years, that remains throughout life at the core of the human psyche. This is the theory I have presented.* How can it be tested? What are its implications?

Testing must proceed from two directions: the brain and the psyche. A bridge must be built using the methods both of neuroscience and psychoanalysis. The key to understanding the brain mechanisms underlying the psyche lies in elucidating the means by which the hippocampus, limbic system, and prefrontal cortex process information and build a behavioral strategy. The research path has in part been traveled. The discovery of the neocortical column, a processing module that acts as a feature detector and, when cascaded in sequence, can perform more and more complex analysis of sensory information, has given neuroscientists an insight into how the entire neocortex may be organized. The same methods of neuroanatomy, neurophysiology, and neurochemistry that have been successfully applied to the sensory neocortex are now being used to study the prefrontal cortex. Columnar organization has been discovered there also. New techniques developed to measure levels of neuron activity in the awake, thinking human brain may help to reveal their function. Despite its complexity, one expects prefrontal cortex function to become much more clear with the course of time.

The methods mentioned above are also currently being used to study the hippocampus. Moreover, several of them, such as the measurement of levels of neuronal activity by means of radioactive tracers or the recording of individual neurons firing via microelectrodes, can be applied while an animal is awake and learning as well as when it is asleep. Thus one can monitor the activity of the hippocampus during these important activities. In addition, one can cut out a slice from the living hippocampus, thus isolating an individual lamella itself, and keep it in a dish, while detailed physiological characteristics are studied. By testing this isolated lamella with known and simple inputs and observing its outputs, one can gain insight into the types of processing that take place in this structural module. Ultimately the logical scheme by which the hippocampus works with the remainder of the limbic system and the neocortex to provide memory consolidation should become apparent.

The route that information takes in passing from neocortex to hippocampus and then to the rest of the limbic system is also being traced slowly and carefully in neuroanatomical studies and by the classical technique of making lesions in certain brain structures and then observing the consequent loss of function. This work is being done in monkeys where loss of memory after specific lesions can be tested, using a number of behavioral tasks. The limbic circuit has been followed functionally, in this manner, from the neocortex, through the hippocampus and the amygdala, to limbic target areas in the thalamus. The next step in functional tracing is the connection to the prefrontal cortex, which is known to exist anatomically.

One line of research that would provide fairly direct data to evaluate the theory I have presented would be to see if the elimination of REM sleep over a period of time, especially before the critical period, interferes with the formulation of species-specific behavioral strategies in lower mammals. The generating mechanism of REM sleep is so complex and so deeply imbedded in the brain stem, however, that no means have yet been found to eliminate it without impairing an animal's behavior. Future understanding of the generating mechanism might allow such means to be found and the experiment to be performed.

Another prospect for testing my theory concerns the echidna. Relatively little study has been devoted to this animal. One could discover whether the echidna truly represented in evolution a new kind of information processing in the mammalian brain by studying its brain, using the same methods that have been applied to study the brains of later mammals. Also, very little is known about the other living monotreme, the duck-billed platypus. Does it show the echidna's unusual neural organization or had nature already implemented the new scheme that we see in later mammals? Again, this question can be answered with today's technology.

Despite its enormous complexity, as a result of these several lines of research, one hopes and expects that in the course of time, measured perhaps in tens of years, the way the brain handles information during waking and sleeping behaviors will be revealed. The theory proposed here will then be confirmed, revised, or supplanted by another in accordance with the new experimental results. The benefit of this research will not simply be the understanding of how the brain governs normal psychological development, but will also provide our best opportunity to alleviate, cure, or prevent mental disease.

What is the role of psychological research in our understanding of the connection between the brain and the psyche? Although I believe that neuroscience can in time reveal the mechanisms of unconscious mental processes, it cannot reveal their content. The keys to the psyche are sleep research in which dream content is recorded and psychoanalysis with dream interpretation by free association. I have reported the rather startling discrepancy between the psychoanalytic expectation that children's dreams would contain the bizarre unconscious material revealed by the psychoanalysis of adults and David Foulkes's finding that this material is largely absent. Sleep research and psychoanalysis should be able to elucidate the questions that have been raised. And my theory has led to a prediction: that despite their apparent dramatic swings from the bizarre to the logical and matter of fact, the content of dreams day by day form a cohesive pattern and reflect each individual's unconscious strategy for survival—his or her unconscious personality. Psychoanalysis is the only discipline that can provide information about this, and indeed analytic findings have led to a concept similar to the one I have suggested here. Jung's observations led him to describe an autonomous entity in the unconscious:

> The active contents of the unconscious do behave in a way I cannot describe better than by the word "autonomous." . . . They have been split off from consciousness and lead a separate existence in the unconscious, being at all times ready to hinder or reinforce the conscious intentions. . . . They always contain memories, wishes, fears, duties, needs or views, with which we have never really come to terms, and for this reason they constantly interfere with our conscious life in a disturbing and usually harmful way.

And Los Angeles psychoanalyst Robert Stoller speaks of his patients as acting according to unconscious "scripts" and presents his views of a separate inner self:

> I suggest that there is still another "self" who, too often, crouches inside the clear-eyed soul and does not intend to change.

Further data are needed. The analytic interpretation of dreams on a day-by-day basis both during psychoanalysis and after, recorded in association with the concurrent events of an individual's life, should provide the necessary information from which theories such as mine may be tested.*

Finally, let us turn back to the objective set out in the introduction: the attempt through the study of the brain to understand man's nature.

We have followed a long evolutionary development of the brain, with the brain and psyche of man as its ultimate result. At its core is the unconscious, the mechanism that formulates and sets strategies for behavior. In lower mammals, this mechanism comprises the total neural system governing behavioral strategy. In humans it is still present; it is the source of neurosis in some and a potent influence on personality and emotion in all.

For those who have questioned the very existence of the unconscious as observed by Freud and later psychoanalysts, my hypothesis affirms that it is indeed real, a product of evolution and the biology of the brain. The concept of the unconscious derived here from brain function is however somewhat different from Freud's. Freud saw the unconscious as containing the id, a caldron of untamed passions and destructive instincts held in check by repression. In contrast, I find the unconscious a cohesive, continually active mental structure which takes note of life's experiences and reacts according to its own scheme of interpretation and responses. This reaction is reflected nightly in our dreams. Though my view of the unconscious is somewhat different from Freud's, I find the unconscious no less important.

To the unconscious core, the heritage from lower species, evolution added in man an unsurpassed intellect, language, and a vast capacity for associative thinking. The result is man's nature, wondrous in the tremendous scope of its intellectual achievement and artistic creativity. But man's nature is flawed, for he endures suffering both from internal disquietude (to use Hippocrates' term) and the irrationality of the society that is his creation.

What are the sources of these flaws? Some can be traced to the unconscious. If the unconscious ideas underlying neurosis and internal conflicts were not locked in place by the mechanism inherited from lower species, they would normally be dispelled by experience and logic. They are, after all, untenable by the light of day. Recalling our earlier example, the father did not literally threaten to castrate his young son; this was only a threat in the child's unconscious thoughts. And for the son, now grown, to stunt and ruin his career, because of the unconscious fear of surpassing his father and his consequent punishment, is at the same time ridiculous and tragic.

What can be done to alleviate or at least diminish this aspect of man's distress? Through psychoanalysis, it is possible for an individual to find the truth of his or her own nature, a source of great satisfaction when it is accomplished. However, the process can only be undertaken by a few, and it may or may not result in a desired behavioral change—a fact I have ascribed to the tenacity of unconscious thought after the critical period. Perhaps of more general value would be the realization by parents of the critical period in childhood development. Unconscious ideas will inevitably become established during the critical period, but every effort can be made to avoid fears of abandonment and other obvious sources of anxiety and conflict.

Lastly, what is the source of man's irrationality in the organization of his society—his wars and the cruelty of his fellowmen? I have said that I do not see the source in a Freudian id filled with destructive repressed instincts. There are clearly sources of violence in the unconscious, which may arise genetically or as a result of early experience. Desires to possess what others have and to eliminate rivals do sit in the unconscious, ready to emerge if life's conditions permit. But in the interests of survival, nature arranged to have such unconscious traits generally modifiable by experience early in life during the critical period. As we have seen, even so basic a trait as a cat killing prey can be modified, so that if the kitten is not given a chance to kill during the critical period, it will never do so easily later in life. Thus, in human beings I see the unconscious engaged primarily in an attempt to adapt during the critical period and beyond. Aggressive drives are present, but they are restrained so as to avoid punishment and insure survival.

Anthropology has offered several possible explanations for man's violence. It has been suggested that there is a genetic inheritance from our primate ancestors to hunt and kill in order to survive, or to defend one's territory, these traits then being passed on in our genes to the next generation. However, any such genetic trait would necessarily have to be expressed through the organization and function of the brain, since the brain controls final behavior, and there is not yet any evidence from neuroscience that this type of inheritance does operate. Further, these hypotheses have been found inadequate by anthropologists themselves on closer inspection of their data.

What then is the source of irrationality and violent behavior within societies and between nations? It appears to lie in the conscious self and its interaction with environmental influences as they are presently constituted. The conscious self is supremely adaptable, easily bent by the forces of society. We are each caught up in the struggle for survival and advancement. To survive, we adopt the rules and mores of society (in our present world, competition within societies as well as between nations), and thus the status quo is perpetuated. The relevant point I wish to draw from the present study of the biological basis of the unconscious is this: Should greater reason prevail and we come to organize our society in a more rational and humane way, our heritage from lower species—our unconscious—will not upset the balance that will have been achieved.

I have proposed a hypothesis. It is only a first step. But ahead along the path of research I believe the objective will be gained; we will finally understand the source of our nature. This knowledge will then be available to be used for our benefit, if we so choose.

Notes and
References

Asterisked notes are the author's comments on the main text. Other notes are bibliographical references.

Chapter 1, Memory, Perception, and Emotion

Page

11 The original report of H.M.'s surgery and its consequences appears in W. B. Scoville and B. Milner, "Loss of Recent Memory after Bilateral Hippocampal Lesions." *Journal of Neurology, Neurosurgery and Psychiatry*, 1957, Vol. 20, p. 11.

12 "Every day is alone . . .": B. Milner, S. Corkin, and H. L. Teuber, "Further Analysis of the Hippocampal Amnesic Syndrome: 14-Year Follow-up Study of H.M." *Neuropsychologia*, 1968, Vol. 6, p. 215.

12 Famous faces test: W. D. Marslen-Wilson and H. L. Teuber, "Memory for Remote Events in Anterograde Amnesia: Recognition of Public Figures from Newsphotographs." *Neuropsychologia*, 1975, Vol. 13, p. 353.

*13 We recall that the amygdala was also removed in H.M. Recent animal research suggests that the amygdala may also have to be removed for the recent memory deficit to be complete. See note 29 for further comments.

13 Wilder Penfield's cases: W. Penfield and B. Milner, "Memory Deficit Produced by Bilateral Lesions of the Hippocampal

Page

Zone." *AMA Archives of Neurology and Psychiatry*, 1958, Vol. 79, p. 475.

*14 With the exception that there may be a long-lasting amnesia for events at about the time of treatment or a month or two beyond it. Unilateral rather than bilateral electroconvulsive shock treatment results in lesser memory disruption and is currently being used in some psychiatric facilities.

14 Squire's memory test utilizing television programs is reported in L. R. Squire, and N. J. Cohen, "Memory and Amnesia: Resistance to Disruption Develops for Years After Learning." *Behavioral and Neural Biology*, 1979, Vol. 25, p. 115.

15 "The data strongly support . . ." ibid.

15 A comprehensive discussion of the processing of long-term memory over a period of several years may be found in L. R. Squire, N. J. Cohen, and L. Nadel, "The Medial Temporal Region and Memory Consolidation: A New Hypothesis," in H. Weingartner and E. Parker, eds., *Memory Consolidation* (Hillsdale, N.J.: Lawrence Erlbaum Associates, 1982).

*16 Seizures are readily induced in the hippocampus by electrical stimulation, and memory disruption may result from such seizures during electroconvulsive shocks. The loss of recent memories may also involve shock effects in the temporal lobe or other parts of the brain.

*16 In addition, H.M.'s intellectual capabilities were virtually unchanged by his surgery; his I.Q. was 112 after the operation compared to 104 before. The Wechsler-Bellevue Intelligence Test was used to measure his general intellectual functioning. This test measures verbal comprehension, vocabulary, and arithmetical skills, and we would expect no change in these capabilities since H.M. retains older memories. As it happens, the questions on this test pertaining to information of events in the past do not ask about recent events (presumably so that the test does not have to be updated periodically), and so the test did not detect H.M.'s memory deficit.

16 Mooney test for hidden faces: Milner, Corkin, and Teuber, op. cit.

17 Mirror drawing test: B. Milner, "Les Troubles de la Memoire Accompagnant des Lesions Hippocampiques Bilaterales,"

Page   *Physiologie de l'Hippocampe* (Paris: Centre National de la
              Recherche Scientifique, 1962).

17   "Tower of Hanoi": N. J. Cohen and S. Corkin, "The Amnesia
      Patient H.M.: Learning and Retention of a Cognitive Skill."
      Society for Neuroscience, 1981, Vol. 7, p. 235.

18   The neuron and its mode of function is described in greater
      detail in C. T. Stevens, "The Neuron," *Scientific American*,
      September 1979.

22   Work of Hubel and Wiesel: For a more complete description
      of the visual system, the nonscientific reader may wish to refer
      to D. H. Hubel, and T. N. Wiesel, "Mechanisms of Vision"
      in the September 1979 issue of *Scientific American*. An excel-
      lent neuroscientific presentation is given in S. W. Kuffler and
      I. G. Nicholls, Part 1, "Neural Organization for Perception"
      in *From Neuron to Brain* (Sunderland, Mass.: Sinauer Asso-
      ciates, Inc., 1976). Hubel and Wiesel were awarded the Nobel
      Prize for their work in 1981.

*23   The angle of our entire visual field as seen by one eye is on the
      order of 150 degrees. The angle covered by one of the circular
      patches is about one half a degree for the part of the scene at
      the center of our gaze.

*23   There are also cells that turn off, cease their random firing,
      when light is focused in the circular area.

24   Multiple striate and prestriate visual regions in the owl mon-
      key: J. F. Baker, S. E. Petersen, W. T. Newsome, and J. M.
      Allman, "Visual Response Properties of Neurons in Four Ex-
      trastriate Visual Areas of the Owl Monkey (Aotus trivirgatus):
      A Quantitative Comparison of Medial, Dorsomedial, Dorso-
      lateral, and Middle Temporal Areas," *Journal of Neurophysiol-
      ogy*, 1981, Vol. 45, p. 397.

26   Experiments concerning neurons in monkey inferotemporal
      cortex that respond to faces are reported in C. G. Gross, C. E.
      Roche-Miranda, and D. B. Bender, "Visual Properties of Neu-
      rons in Inferotemporal Cortex of the Macaque," *Journal of
      Neurophysiology*, 1972, Vol. 35, p. 96, and D. F. Perrett,
      E. T. Rolls, and W. Caan, "Visual Neurons Responsive to
      Faces in the Monkey Temporal Cortex," *Experimental Brain
      Research*, 1982, Vol. 47, p. 329.

26   The failure following neocortical lesions to recognize single

Page

           perceptional categories is documented in Chapter 3, J. Konorski, *Integrative Activity of the Brain* (Chicago: Chicago University Press, 1967).

*27   The anatomy and workings of the cortical column are just beginning to be unraveled. The boundaries of the column are not precisely defined since the feature extraction properties, such as line orientation, shift gradually in adjacent columns of neurons. The concept of the cortical column is discussed in depth by V. B. Mountcastle in G. M. Edelman and V. B. Mountcastle, *The Mindful Brain: Cortical Organization and Group Selective Theory of Higher Function* (Cambridge, Mass.: MIT Press, 1978).

27   Cortical columnar organization in the motor cortex has been found by Hiroshi Asanuma of the Rockefeller University and in prefrontal cortex by Patricia Goldman-Rakic of Yale University.

*28   As an example, H.M. is able to solve the puzzle of the Tower of Hanoi by many acts of trial and error, much as a normal individual does, although he cannot remember any given act or even the fact that he has worked at the puzzle at all. In H.M. and in normals, the strategy devised to master the problem is apparently established in the neocortex over repeated trials.

29   The anatomical evidence that neocortical inputs arising from sensory associational areas converge in entorhinal cortex to constitute the major input to the hippocampus is summarized in G. W. Van Hoesen, "The Parahippocampal Gyrus—New Observations Regarding Its Cortical Connections in the Monkey." *Trends in Neuroscience,* October 1982, p. 345, Elsevier Biomedical Press. In man and monkeys the entorhinal cortex is located in the parahippocampal gyrus, a part of the temporal lobe lying next to the hippocampus.

*29   Along with the studies of memory deficits in patients like H.M., there have been many attempts to reproduce these deficits in animals by the surgical removal of the hippocampus, the amygdala, or both. These experiments have been made difficult by the obvious fact that the animal cannot be asked directly whether or not it recalls a given object or event. Instead the animal is required to carry out an action within a given test situation from which memory or the lack of it is implied. A commonly used memory test for monkeys is the following: The monkey is presented with a small object—a child's toy or a block, for example—which covers a shallow well in a table in front of it. In the well, hidden beneath the object, is a food reward such as a peanut, which the animal can pick up and eat after lifting the object. Following a delay of some period of time, say 10 seconds, the animal is presented with two objects, the old one and a new and different one, each covering a well. The peanut reward is beneath the new object—that is, the monkey is rewarded for choosing an object it has never seen before. Animals rapidly learn to perform this task almost perfectly. After this training, monkeys have been operated on and their hippocampus removed bilaterally. They were no longer able to perform the task, but could relearn it in a normal number of trials. H.M.'s syndrome was not reproduced, despite complete lesioning of the hippocampus. Removal of the amygdala yielded a similar result; the task was forgotten but could be relearned in normal fashion.

It will be recalled that in H.M., Scoville had removed both the hippocampus and amygdala bilaterally. In 1978, Mishkin duplicated this more extensive surgery in monkeys. The ability to perform the task was indeed lost, establishing a correspondence to H.M. The tentative suggestion at that time was that, in some way, despite the totally different anatomical and neural organization of the hippocampus and amygdala, one structure could substitute for the other in processing memory.

New experiments in the Mishkin laboratory now suggest a more refined neural logic. Hippocampal damage alone does indeed produce a memory deficit: The monkey cannot recall the position of an object on the table (whether it is on the left or right). Amygdala damage alone also produces a subtle deficit of a different type. In all, the interaction of hippocampus and amygdala in processing memory are not yet understood, but the findings of these lesion experiments are compatible with the concept suggested in this chapter. If the animal with a hippocampus but no amygdala could be asked why it consistently chose the novel object, it might reply that it remembered doing that before, although it might not recall the plea-

Page

sure of the reward (the event was recalled but not the emotional association). The animal with an amygdala but no hippocampus would say that it chose the novel object because, although it did not remember carrying out such a procedure previously, the new object (analyzed and identified in the temporal neocortex) was associated in its mind (via the amygdala) with the pleasure of a food reward. The animal with neither hippocampus nor amygdala would have no remembrance of the event nor an affective association to it and would have no way to reestablish the connection between the novel object and reward. The monkey would therefore neither remember nor be able to relearn the task. Mishkin's work is reviewed in M. Mishkin, L. G. Ungerleider, and K. A. Macko, "Object Vision and Spatial Vision: Two Cortical Pathways," *Trends in Neuroscience*, October 1983, p. 414, and in M. Mishkin, "A Memory System in the Monkey," *Philosophic Transactions of the Royal Society*, London, 1982, B 298, p. 85.

30   P. D. McLean, "Some Psychiatric Implications of Physiological Studies of Frontotemporal Portion of Limbic System (Visceral Brain)" *Electroencephalography and Clinical Neurophysiology*, 1952, Vol. 4, p. 407.

31   J. W. Papez, "A Proposed Mechanism of Emotion," *Archives of Neurology and Psychiatry*, 1937, Vol. 38, p. 725.

*31   Papez's proposed mechanism was the following: "It is thus evident that the afferent pathways from the receptor organs split at the thalamic level into three routes, each conducting a stream of impulses of special importance. One route conducts impulses through the . . . thalamus . . . to the corpus striatum [the basal ganglia, a group of subcortical nuclei associated with action or movement]. This route represents 'the stream of movement.' The second conducts impulses from the thalamus . . . to the lateral cerebral cortex. This route represents 'the stream of thought.' The third conducts a set of concomitant impulses through the . . . thalamus by way of the mammillary body and the anterior thalamic nuclei to the gyrus cinguli, in the medial wall of the cerebral hemisphere. This route represents 'the stream of feeling.' In this way, the sensory excitations which reach the lateral cortex . . . receive their emotional coloring from the concurrent processes of hy-

Page   pothalamic origin which irradiate them from the gyrus
                cinguli."

32   H. Klüver and P. C. Bucy, "Preliminary Analysis of Functions
     of the Temporal Lobes in Monkeys," *Archives of Neurology
     and Psychiatry,* 1939, Vol. 42, p. 979.

Chapter 2, Sleep and Dreaming

35   Kleitman's early experiments are described in Nathaniel
     Kleitman, *Sleep and Wakefulness* (Chicago: University of Chi-
     cago Press, 1963).

38   Confirmation of Berger rhythm: E. D. Adrian and B. H. C.
     Mathews, "Berger Rhythm: Potential Changes from Occipital
     Lobes in Man," *Brain,* 1934, Vol. 57, p. 355.

38   Neocortical origin of alpha rhythm: E. D. Adrian and K.
     Yamagiwa, "The Origin of the Berger Rhythm," *Brain,* 1935,
     Vol. 58, p. 323.

40   "Stumbled" into it, Kleitman, op. cit., p. 92.

40   Rapid eye movements in infants: E. Aserinsky and N.
     Kleitman, "Two Types of Ocular Motility Occurring in
     Sleep," *Journal of Applied Psychology,* 1955, Vol. 8, p. 1.

40   Motility cycle in infants: E. Aserinsky and N. Kleitman, "A
     Motility Cycle in Sleeping Infants as Manifested by Ocular
     and Gross Bodily Activity," *Journal of Applied Psychology,*
     1955, Vol. 8, p. 11.

41   First study of REM sleep in adults, "To test this supposition
     . . .": E. Aserinsky and N. Kleitman, "Regularly Occurring
     Periods of Eye Motility, and Concomitant Phenomena during
     Sleep," *Science,* 1953, Vol. 118, p. 273. (This study in adults
     was performed later than the study in infants. The publication
     of the experiment in infants was apparently delayed.)

42   Dement study: W. Dement and N. Kleitman, "Cyclic Varia-
     tions in EEG during Sleep and their Relation of Eye Move-
     ments, Body Motility and Dreaming," *Electroencepha-
     lography and Clinical Neurophysiology,* 1957, Vol. 9, p. 673.

44   Dement experiment in the cat: W. Dement, "The Occur-

Page   rence of Low Voltage, Fast Electroencephalogram Patterns During Behavioral Sleep in the Cat," *Electroencephalography and Clinical Neurophysiology*, 1958, Vol. 10, p. 291.

46   Activity of neurons in neocortex during REM sleep: E. V. Evarts, "Visual Cortex Neurons in Cat as Active During REM as During Waking with Visual Stimulation," in G. C. Quarton, T. Melnechuk, and F. O. Schmitt, eds., *The Neurosciences* (New York: The Rockefeller University Press, 1967), p. 545.

46   Jouvet's work is described in the chapter "Neurophysiology of the States of Sleep," op. cit., p. 529.

47   Brain-stem lesions result in active behavior during REM sleep: M. Jouvet, op. cit. Also see A. R. Morrison, "Brain-Stem Regulation of Behavior During Sleep and Wakefulness," in James M. Sprague and Alan N. Epstein, eds., *Progress in Psychobiology and Physiological Psychology*, Vol. 8 (New York: Academic Press, 1979), p. 91, and A. R. Morrison, "A Window on the Sleeping Brain," *Scientific American*, April 1983.

*47   The question naturally arises whether sleepwalking in humans is caused by a loss of inhibition of motor centers during REM sleep, similar to the phenomenon seen in cats with their inhibitory centers destroyed. This is not the case however. Sleepwalking occurs predominantly during stage 4 of sleep (a non-REM period), or upon awakening from stage 4. Its physiological basis is not known, but sleepwalking does not appear to be related to REM sleep or to dreaming. The subject is discussed in R. J. Broughton, "Sleep Disorders: Disorders of Arousal?" *Science*, 1968, Vol. 159, p. 1070.

48   REM deprivation experiment: W. Dement, "The Effect of Dream Deprivation," *Science*, 1960, Vol. 131, p. 1705.

49   Mentation during sleep onset: D. Foulkes and G. Vogel, "Mental Activity at Sleep Onset," *Journal of Abnormal Psychology*, 1965, Vol. 70, p. 231.

49   Mentation during non-REM sleep: This work is summarized in Chapter 4 of David Foulkes, *The Psychology of Sleep* (New York: Charles Scribner's Sons, 1966).

50   "On those nights . . .": A. Rechtschaffen, G. Vogel, and G. Shaikun, "Interrelatedness of Mental Activity During Sleep," *Archives of General Psychiatry*, 1963, Vol. 9, p. 536.

Page   51   Development of sleep over the life span: H. P. Roffwarg, J. N. Muzio, and W. C. Dement, "Ontogenetic Development of the Human Sleep-dream Cycle," *Science*, 1966, Vol. 152, p. 604.

*53   It is also conceivable that REM sleep fulfills two functions, one during early development and a second thereafter.

53   Sleep in various mammals is described in the article T. Allison and H. Van Twyver, "The Evolution of Sleep," *Natural History*, 1970, Vol. 79, p. 56.

54   Sleep in the echidna: T. Allison, H. Van Twyver, and W. R. Goff, "Electrophysiological Studies of the Echidna, Tachyglossus aculeatus, I: Waking and Sleep," *Archives of Italian Biology*, 1972, Vol. 110, p. 145. A book giving a comprehensive description of the echidna is Mervyn Griffiths, *The Biology of the Monotremes* (New York: Academic Press, 1978).

55   Increase of slow-wave sleep after marathons: C. M. Shapiro, R. Bortz, D. Mitchell, P. Bartel, and P. Jooste, "Slow-wave Sleep: A Recovery Period After Exercise," *Science*, 1981, Vol. 214, p. 1253.

56   Growth hormone: Y. Takahaski, "Growth Hormone Secretion Related to the Sleep and Waking Rhythm," in R. Drucker-Colín, M. Shkurovich, and M. B. Sterman, eds., *The Functions of Sleep* (New York: Academic Press, 1971).

56   Prefrontal cortex of echidna investigated electrophysiologically: T. Allison and W. R. Goff, "Electrophysiological Studies of the Echidna, Tachyglossus aculeatus, III: Sensory and Interhemispheric Evoked Potentials," *Archives of Italian Biology*, 1972, Vol. 110, p. 195.

56   Prefrontal cortex of echidna defined by connections to mediodorsal nucleus of the thalamus: Wally Welker and Richard A. Lende, "Thalamocortical Relationships in Echidna (Tachyglossus aculeatus)," Chapter 15 in Sven O. E. Ebbeson, ed., *Comparative Neurology of the Telencephalon* (New York, London: Plenum Press, 1980).

56   "The most obtrusive feature . . .": G. Elliot Smith, "Mammalia, order Monotremata," In Catalogue of the Physiological Series of Comparative Anatomy, Vol. 2, 2nd ed. Museum of

Page   the Royal College of Surgeons, London, England, 1902, p.
                138.

59   "The most crucial constituents . . . ," Joaquin M. Fuster,
      The Prefrontal Cortex (New York: Raven Press, 1980), p. 128.

59   ". . . do not evaluate . . . ," quoted in A. R. Luria, *Higher
      Cortical Functions in Man* (New York: Basic Books, 1966), p.
      222. This book presents a broad study of disturbances of func-
      tion following lesions of various regions of the neocortex in
      man.

Chapter 3, The Early Discoveries

For the reader desiring a more comprehensive account of
Freud's life and work, reference should be made to Ernest
Jones, *The Life and Work of Sigmund Freud,* Vols. I, II, and
III (New York: Basic Books, 1955), hereafter referred to as
Jones. An informative recent biography is Ronald W. Clark,
Freud, the Man and the Cause (New York: Random House,
1980), referred to as *Clark.* Freud's complete works appear in
the twenty-four-volume series, *The Standard Edition of the
Complete Psychological Works of Sigmund Freud,* edited by
James Strachey (London: Hogarth Press, 1953), referred to
below as *Standard Edition.* In addition, the French historian
Henri F. Ellenberger has written a definitive history of the
development of psychiatry, *The Discovery of the Unconscious*
(New York: Basic Books, 1970), referred to hereafter as *Ellenberger,* which I recommend to the interested reader.

67   "I am coming with money . . . ," Freud–Martha Bernays
      correspondence, June 20, 1885, in Ernest L. Freud, ed., *Let-
      ters of Sigmund Freud, 1873–1939* (New York: Basic Books,
      1975), p. 154.

67   The case of Anna O. was described by Breuer in *Studies on
      Hysteria* (1893–1895), which constitutes Vol. II of *Standard
      Edition.* A perceptive analysis of the case of Anna O., put in
      the context of cases of a similar nature reported earlier, is
      given in *Ellenberger,* p. 480.

Page   68   "For two weeks . . . ," *Standard Edition*, Vol. II, p. 25.

69   "She was carried back . . . ," *Standard Edition*, Vol. II, p. 33.

70   "These findings . . . ," *Standard Edition*, Vol. II, p. 35.

70   Anna O. took some time to recover her full mental balance: Frank J. Solloway, *Freud, Biologist of the Mind* (New York: Basic Books, 1979), p. 84.

71   Decline and change in nature of hysteria: *Ellenberger*, pp. 256, 480.

72   As Freud stated later: *Jones*, Vol. I, p. 233.

72   "I received the profoundest impression . . . ," *Standard Edition*, Vol. XX, p. 17.

73   "Charcot, who is one of the . . . ," Freud–Martha Bernays correspondence, November 24, 1885, op. cit., p. 184.

73   "For twenty-five centuries . . . ," *Ellenberger*, p. 142.

75   "In the normal state . . . ," ibid., p. 130.

76   *The Three Faces of Eve* by Corbett H. Thigpen and Harvey M. Cleckley (New York: McGraw-Hill Book Co., 1957).

76   Daniel Keyes, *The Minds of Billy Milligan* (New York: Random House, 1981).

77   Coaching of Charcot's patients: *Ellenberger*, pp. 97–100.

78   "Unluckily I was soon . . . ," *Standard Edition*, Vol. II, p. 16.

79   "degrades a human being," *Jones*, Vol. I, p. 235.

80   "The therapeutic success . . . ," *Standard Edition*, Vol. II, p. 101.

80   "This was the method . . . ," *Jones*, Vol. I, p. 243.

82   "If we subject . . . a source of the Nile of neuropathology," "The Aetiology of Hysteria," in Philip Rieff, ed., *Early Psychoanalytic Writings* (New York: Collier Books, 1963), pp. 177–187. Also in *Collected Papers of Sigmund Freud* (New York: Basic Books, 1959), pp. 185–239.

84   "But I may also . . ." Rieff, op. cit., p. 194.

85   "I have now come to the end . . ." ibid., p. 203.

86   "With a beating heart . . ." *Clark*, p. 134.

86   "We have arrived at our opinions . . ." Rieff, "On the Theory of Hysterical Attacks," op. cit., p. 29.

87   "Indeed, the more we . . ." ibid., p. 44.

87   "I regard this distinction . . ." *Standard Edition*, Vol. II, p. 286.

Page   87   "You might think . . ." Rieff, "The Aetiology of Hysteria,"
                  op. cit., p. 181.

           88   "It is self-evident . . ." *Standard Edition*, Vol. II, p. 246.

           89   "The case of Anna O. . . ." quoted in Paul F. Crainfield,
                  "Josef Breuer's Evaluation of His Contribution of Psycho-
                  analyses," *The International Journal of Psycho-Analyses*. Vol.
                  XXXIX, Part V, 1958, p. 2.

           89   "I was at last obliged . . ." *Standard Edition*, Vol. XX, p. 34.

           90   "Analysis had led back . . ." *Standard Edition*, Vol. XIV, p.
                  17.

Chapter 4, **The Interpretation of Dreams**

           91   "I myself found it . . ." *Standard Edition*, Vol. XXII, p. 7.

           92   "In self-analysis the danger . . ." *Standard Edition*, Vol.
                  XXII, p. 234.

           93   "In the following pages . . ." Quotations from *The Interpre-
                  tation of Dreams* are taken from *The Basic Writings of
                  Sigmund Freud*, translated and edited by A. A. Brill (New
                  York: Random House, Modern Library, 1938), hereafter re-
                  ferred to as IOD. This quotation appears on p. 183.

           95   "A great hall . . ." ibid. p. 196.

           96   "Nevertheless . . ." ibid. p. 197.

           96   "I cannot help . . ." ibid. p. 202.

           97   "Here the reproach of rashness . . ." ibid. p. 204.

           97   "Another reproach directed . . ." ibid. p. 204.

           97   "For the result of the dream is . . ." ibid. p. 205.

           98   "I do not wish to assert . . ." ibid. p. 206.

           98   "My friend Leopold . . ." ibid. p. 200.

           99   "How on earth . . ." This passage has been taken from the
                  translation of *The Interpretation of Dreams* by James Strachey.
                  Standard Edition, Vol. IV, p. 115.

           99   "In the dream . . ." IOD, p. 203.

          100   "I am making fun of Dr. M. . . ." ibid. p. 202.

          101   Erik H. Erikson, "The Dream Specimen of Psychoanalysis,"

Page   *Journal of the American Psychoanalytic Association*, 1954, Vol. 2, p. 5.

102   "Then when I was seven . . ." IOD, p. 274.

102   "In the sexual constitution . . ." ibid., p. 234.

103   "But how is it possible . . ." ibid., p. 446.

104   "mark of the beast . . ." ibid., p. 251.

104   "A number of children . . ." ibid., p. 301.

105   "But how does the childish . . ." ibid., p. 301.

106   "I had the opportunity . . ." ibid., p. 306.

107   "At this point, an admonition . . ." ibid., p. 505.

*109   By a previous marriage, Freud's father, Jacob, had two grown sons, Philipp and Emanuel, aged twenty and twenty-four, at the time of Freud's birth.

112   "There is a terrible storm . . ." ibid., p. 398.

113   "I am walking in the street . . ." ibid., p. 376.

118   "Project for a Scientific Psychology," *Standard Edition*, Vol. I, p. 283.

119   Schur's paper, including the relevant Freud–Fliess correspondence and his commentary, appears in R. M. Loewenstein, L. M. Newman, M. Schur, and A. J. Solnit, eds., *Psychoanalysis—A General Psychology* (New York: International Universities Press, 1966). Letters of Freud–Fliess correspondence identified by date. Quotation "But it was not only his . . ." appears on p. 70.

Chapter 5, Later Developments

127   "many details . . ." quoted in *Clark*, p. 81.

128   "sounded like a . . ." *Ellenberger*, p. 448.

129   "Good hearted and considerate . . ." *Clark*, p. 218.

129   "The meetings of the Vienna . . ." Abram Kardiner, *My Analysis with Freud* (New York: W. W. Norton, 1977), p. 85, hereafter called *Kardiner*.

130   "In the meanwhile . . ." ibid., p. 56.

133   "This is the first . . ." *Jones*, Vol. II, p. 57.

*133   In Freud's words, written in 1894: "I should like finally to

Page

dwell for a moment on the hypothesis which I have made use of in the exposition of the defense neuroses. I mean the conception that among the psychic functions there is something which should be differentiated (an amount of affect, a sum of excitation), something having all the attributes of a quantity—although we possess no means of measuring it—a something which is capable of increase, decrease, displacement and discharge, and which extended itself over the memory traces of an idea like an electric charge over the surface of the body. We can apply this hypothesis, which by the way already underlies our theory of 'abreaction' in the same sense as the physicist employs the conception of a fluid electric current. For the present it is justified by its utility in correlating and explaining diverse psychical conditions." Rieff, "The Defense Neuro-psychosis," op. cit., p. 80.

135   "endeavoring to master . . ." *Standard Edition*, Vol. XVIII, p. 32.

136   "The ego after all . . ." *Standard Edition*, Vol. XIX, p. 25.

137   "Scientifically I still do not . . ." quoted by *Clark*, p. 294.

139   All letters are contained in *The Freud–Jung Letters: The Correspondence Between Sigmund Freud and C. G. Jung*, edited by Wm. McGuire, Bollingen Series XCIV (Princeton, N.J.: Princeton University Press, 1974).

142   "Freud points to the . . ." C. G. Jung, *Critique of Psychoanalysis*, Bollingen Series XX (Princeton, N.J.: Princeton University Press, 1975), p. 23.

143   "We deceive ourselves . . ." ibid., p. 25.

143   "This kind of . . ." ibid.

143   "The term Oedipus complex . . ." ibid., p. 70.

144   "The ultimate and deepest . . ." ibid., p. 101.

144   "I do not doubt . . ." ibid., p. 228.

147   "Freudian psychology had flooded . . ." quoted by Christopher Lasch in "Sacrificing Freud," New York *Times Magazine*, February 22, 1976, p. 70.

148   "Once he located . . ." *Kardiner*, p. 84.

149   "Freud's perspective . . ." ibid., p. 99.

*150   For expositions and further discussions of ego psychology, see Anna Freud, *The Ego and the Mechanisms of Defense* (New York: International Universities Press, 1946), Erik H. Erikson,

Page   *Childhood and Society* (New York: W.W. Norton and Company, 1950), and Heinz Hartmann, *Ego Psychology and the Problem of Adaptation* (New York: International Universities Press, 1958).

*153   This was necessarily the case in psycho-history, the psychoanalytic interpretation of the lives of public figures. These figures might not be alive. Alive or not, they were being analyzed without the benefit of psychoanalytic material originating directly from them.

153   "One is therefore led . . ." Sidney Hook, ed., *Psychoanalysis, Scientific Method and Philosophy* (New York: Grove Press, 1959), p. 44.

153   "The two psychoanalytic theories . . . ," Karl R. Popper, *Conjectures and Refutations: The Growth of Scientific Knowledge* (New York: Basic Books, 1962), p. 37.

155   "Psychoanalysis has innumerable . . . ," Emanuel Peterfreund and Jacob T. Schwartz, *Information, Systems, and Psychoanalysis* (New York: International Universities Press, 1971), p. 84.

*155   Richard M. Jones, *The New Psychology of Dreaming* (New York: Grune and Stratton, 1970) contains a comprehensive summary of dream theories.

156   The study of homosexuality appears in Irving Bieber, ed., *Homosexuality, A Psychoanalytic Study of Male Homosexuals* (New York: Basic Books, 1962).

156   Two leading lines of research are described in Margaret S. Mahler, Fred Pine, and Anni Bergman, *The Psychological Birth of the Human Infant* (New York: Basic Books, 1975), and John Bowlby, "Psychoanalysis as a Natural Science," *The International Review of Psychoanalysis*, 1981, Vol. 8, p. 243.

*156   Such attempts have been made through the years. The endeavor has always been limited by the state of knowledge of the physical workings of the brain. Freud abandoned his own effort, *Project for a Scientific Psychology (Standard Edition*, Vol. I), when he saw that the neurophysiology of his day did not provide an adequate basis for a theory. The status of the brain-psyche connection was summarized in 1953 by psychoanalyst Lawrence Kubie in "Some Implications for Psychoanalysis of Modern Concepts of the Organization of the Brain," which appeared in the *Psychoanalytic Quarterly*, Vol.

Page   XXII (1953), p. 21. A coherent synthesis was not possible at
                that time. Two recent articles suggest that knowledge in
                neuroscience may have advanced to the stage where the brain-
                psyche linkage may be fruitfully explored. The first is a broad
                review of psychoanalytic research, Peter Fonagy, "The Inte-
                gration of Psychoanalysis and Experimental Science," *The In-
                ternational Review of Psychoanalysis*, 1982, Vol. 9, p. 125.
                The second is an analysis of the possible neurophysiological
                basis of anxiety by neuroscientist Eric Kandel, "From Meta-
                psychology to Molecular Biology: Explorations into the Nature
                of Anxiety," *The American Journal of Psychiatry*, 1983, Vol.
                140:10, p. 1277.

157   Survey of East Coast Analysts, cited in Seymour Fisher and
                Roger R. Greenberg, "The Scientific Evaluation of Freud's
                Theories and Therapy," *A Book of Readings*, Vol. II (New
                York: Basic Books, 1978), p. 299. This work is a two-volume
                study surveying various attempts to evaluate Freudian theory
                and practice utilizing psychological tests and interviews of
                both patients and analysts. I recommend Vol. I to the reader
                desiring more detailed information in this area.

159   "One has the impression . . ." *Standard Edition*, Vol. XXII,
                p. 228.

159   Bruno Bettelheim, "Freud and the Soul," *The New Yorker*,
                March 1, 1982.

159   "Freud showed us how . . ." ibid., p. 52.

Chapter 6, Critical Period

162   Imprinting: for a definitive discussion, see P. R. Marler, R. J.
                Dooling, and S. Zoloth, "Comparative Perspectives on Ethol-
                ogy and Behavioral Development," Chapter 6 in Marc H.
                Bornstein, ed., *Comparative Methods in Psychology* (Hillsdale,
                N.J.: Lawrence Erlbaum Associates, 1980).

166   Categorical perception: These experiments are described in
                W. Strange and J. J. Jenkins, "The Role of Language Experi-
                ence in the Perception of Speech," in R. D. Walk and H. J.

Page   Pick, eds., *Perception and Experience* (New York: Plenum Press, 1978). The reader should also refer to Peter D. Eimes and Joanne L. Miller, "Effects of Selective Adaptation on the Perception of Speech and Visual Patterns: Evidence for Feature Detectors," in the same volume.

167   Studies of categorical perception in Japanese people appear in H. Goto, "Auditory Perception by Normal Japanese Adults of the Sounds 'L' and 'R,' " *Neuropsychologica*, 1971, Vol. 9, p. 317.

168   Acquisition of language: A comprehensive account is given by Eric Lenneburg, *Biological Foundations of Language* (New York: John Wiley and Sons, 1967).

169   Hubel and Wiesel reported on the experiments they performed in young kittens in the following papers: D. H. Hubel, and T. N. Wiesel, "Receptive Fields of Cells in Striate Cortex of Very Young, Visually Inexperienced Kittens," *Journal of Neurophysiology*, 1963, Vol. 26, p. 994; "Single-Cell Responses in Striate Cortex of Kittens Deprived of Vision in One Eye," *Journal of Neurophysiology*, 1963, Vol. 26, p. 1003; "The Period of Susceptibility to the Physiological Effects of Unilateral Eye Closure in Kittens," *Journal of Physiology*, 1970, Vol. 226, p. 419.

171   "As an animal walked . . ." Wiesel and Hubel, in "Single-Cell Responses . . . ," op. cit., p. 1006.

172   Kittens raised seeing only vertical or horizontal lines: C. Blakemore and G. F. Cooper, "Development of the Brain Depends on the Visual Environment," *Nature*, 1970, Vol. 228, p. 477.

173   H. V. B. Hirsch and D. N. Spinelli, "Visual Experience Modifies Distribution of Horizontally and Vertically Oriented Receptive Fields in Cats," *Science*, 1970, Vol. 168, p. 869.

174   Astigmatism: D. E. Mitchell, R. D. Freeman, M. Millodot, and G. Haegerstrom, "Meridional Amblyopia: Evidence for Modification of the Human Visual System by Early Visual Experience," *Vision Research*, 1973, Vol. 13, p. 535.

174   In his book, *Cat Behavior* (New York, London: Garland Press, 1979) Paul Leyhausen has meticulously reported many behavioral observations of a number of cat species both in normal and experimental conditions.

174   "Both young and old . . ." ibid., p. 64.

Page   175   "Young domestic cats . . ." ibid., p. 65.

176   "When the kitten is about . . ." ibid., p. 81.

177   "The peak of readiness to kill . . ." ibid., p. 92.

178   "The most important role . . ." ibid., p. 75.

*179   This is a very active field of research. Synaptic facilitation lasting for hours and perhaps days has been found in the hippocampus after a neuronal circuit is activated repetitively. Gary Lynch and associates at the University of California at Irvine have identified a mechanism operating at the synapse that appears to be responsible for the facilitation. Long-lasting synaptic facilitation has also been found in the nervous system of the sea snail Aplysia by Eric Kandel and colleagues at Columbia University. The mechanism here is different from that in the hippocampus. Nature may have provided many means by which repetitive use of a neural pathway enhances subsequent transmission of a signal along the same pathway.

Chapter 7, Hippocampal Theta Rhythm

180   Description of Green and Arduini experiment: J. D. Green and A. A. Arduini, "Hippocampal Electrical Activity in Arousal," *Journal of Neurophysiology,* 1954, Vol. 17, p. 533.

182   "A train of sinusoidal . . ." ibid., p. 538.

183   Species-specific behavioral correlates of theta rhythm: J. Winson, "Interspecies Differences in the Occurrence of Theta," *Behavioral Biology,* 1972, Vol. 7, p. 479. For a review of theta rhythm in various species see T. E. Robinson, "Hippocampal Rhythmic Slow-Wave Activity (RSA; Theta): A Critical Analysis of Selected Studies and Discussion of Possible Species-Differences," *Brain Research Reviews,* 1980, Vol. 2, p. 69.

*186   Although correct in its essentials, this flow of information is complicated by a number of factors. Not only does the input to the lamella from the neocortex reach the first stage of the hippocampal circuit, but a portion of the input also reaches the third stage directly without traversing the three-stage circuit. However, this secondary input is oddly ineffective. There

Page   is undoubtedly some behavioral condition in which it is active, but it cannot be activated by electrical stimulation in anesthetized animals.

There are other inputs to all three stages of the circuit. There is one input from the septum, a structure through which information of an emotional or affective nature arising in the amygdala (as mentioned in Chapter 1) may reach the hippocampus. There are several inputs from the lower brain, as will be described in the next chapter, and sites within the lamella where hormones may act. The hippocampi are paired structures, one on the left and one on the right. Left and right hippocampi are interconnected with a series of pathways, and the lamellae are believed to be connected one to another by pathways running parallel to the long axis of the hippocampus, perpendicular to the plane of the lamella.

On the level of neurons, there are three principal types of neurons, each associated with one of the stages of processing. These neurons are supplemented by dozens of types of interneurons—neurons whose dendrites and axons do not leave the hippocampus but carry out internal processing within the three-stage and longitudinal circuits. Lastly, each of the principal neurons is an immensely complicated neural machine, integrating thousands of synaptic inputs and either transmitting a series of action potentials or not according to its own logic. Thus, despite its rather simple hookup of three main cell groups, the hippocampal lamella is a complex processing unit whose function and mode of operation is unknown. However, the contributions the hippocampus makes to our understanding of psychological function can be derived from the knowledge we do have of theta rhythm and the path of information flow through the three-stage hippocampal circuit.

187   Intracellular recording of theta rhythm: S. E. Fox, S. Wolfson, and J. B. Ranck, "Investigation of the Mechanisms of Hippocampal Theta Rhythm: Approaches and Prospects," in W. Seifert, ed., *Neurobiology of the Hippocampus* (New York: Academic Press, 1983), p. 303.

*188   This occurred in the following way. The internal currents which constituted the theta rhythm were electrically biasing the neurons cyclically. During one phase of the theta rhythm

Page

(for example the peak) the bias was such that the signal arriving along the three-stage circuit was transmitted. At all other times the signal was relatively restricted.

188   I have described these experiments in the following papers: J. Winson, "Patterns of Hippocampal Theta Rhythm in the Freely Moving Rat," *Electroencephalography and Clinical Neurophysiology*, 1974, Vol. 36, p. 291; "Hippocampal Theta Rhythm. I. Depth Profiles in the Curarized Rat," *Brain Research*, 1976, Vol. 103, p. 57; "Hippocampal Theta Rhythm. II. Depth Profiles in the Freely Moving Rabbit," *Brain Research*, 1976, Vol. 103, p. 71.

189   Theta rhythm also generated in entorhinal cortex: S. J. Mitchell and J. B. Ranck, "Generation of Theta Rhythm in Medial Entorhinal Cortex of Freely Moving Rats," *Brain Research*, 1980, Vol. 189, p. 49.

*189   How the brain manages to turn on theta rhythm only during certain behaviors is a subject of considerable interest in which only a small amount of progress has been made. Somewhere in the brain, behavior must be monitored, and there must be a mechanism to initiate theta rhythm only during particular species-specific activities. This may occur in the brain stem, or higher up in the circuits leading to the hippocampus. Indeed the very circuits that initiate the behavior may start the rhythm. In any case, the system that generates theta rhythm seems to be genetically prewired somewhat differently in each species.

Brain-stem generation of theta rhythm is reviewed in R. P. Vertes, "Brain Stem Generation of Hippocampal EEG" in G. A. Kerkut and J. W. Phillis, eds., *Progress in Neurobiology*, Vol. 19 (Elmsford, N.Y.: Pergamon Press, 1982), p. 159. Case Vanderwolf and his colleagues have separated two components of the theta-generating system that govern theta rhythm during movement and sensory stimulation without movement (as in the rabbit), respectively, using pharmacological methods. This is reported in "Reticulo-Cortical Activity and Behavior: A Critique of the Arousal Theory and a New Synthesis," *The Behavioral and Brain Sciences*, 1981, Vol. 5, p. 459.

*190   Foteos Macrides of the Worcester Foundation for Experimental Biology and Howard Eichenbaum of Wellesley College

Page   have trained rats to discriminate odor and respond by holding
their noses in a small hole. The rats, kept slightly thirsty, are
rewarded with water when they learn to detect a particular
odor and perform the task. At this time the inhalation, firing
of sensory neurons in the olfactory bulb, and vibrissae movement are all precisely linked to the theta rhythm. See F.
Macrides, H. B. Eichenbaum, and W. B. Forbes, "Temporal
Relationship Between Sniffing and the Limbic Theta Rhythm
During Odor Discrimination Reversal Learning," *The Journal
of Neuroscience*, 1982, Vol. 2, p. 1705. The theory of the role
of theta rhythm in synchronizing sensory input was first enunciated by Barry Komisaruk of Rutgers University. The theory
is reviewed in B. R. Komisaruk, "The Role of Rhythmical
Brain Activity in Sensorimotor Integration," in James M.
Sprague and Allan N. Epstein, eds., *Progress in Psychobiology
and Physiological Integration* (New York: Academic Press,
1977), Vol. 7.

Chapter 8, Neuronal Gating in the Hippocampus

193   Characteristics of norepinephrine containing neurons of locus
coeruleus: G. Aston-Jones and F. E. Bloom, "Norepinephrine-
containing Locus Coeruleus Neurons in Behaving Rats Exhibit Pronounced Response to Non-noxious Environmental
Stimuli," *Journal of Neuroscience*, 1981, Vol. 1, p. 887; G.
Aston-Jones and F. E. Bloom, "Norepinephrine-containing
Locus Coeruleus Neurons in Behaving Rats Anticipate Fluctu-
ations in the Sleep-waking Cycle," *Journal of Neuroscience*,
1981, Vol. 1, p. 876.

196   This experiment is described in the following papers by J.
Winson and C. Abzug: "Gating of Neuronal Transmission in
the Hippocampus: Efficacy of Transmission Varies with Be-
havioral State," *Science*, 1977, Vol. 196, p. 1223; "Neuronal
Transmission Through Hippocampal Pathways Dependent on
Behavior," *Journal of Neurophysiology*, 1978, Vol. 41, p. 716;
"Dependence upon Behavior of Neuronal Transmission from

Page   Perforant Pathway through Entorhinal Cortex," *Brain Research*, 1978, Vol. 147, p. 422.

*197   Experiments of this sort were first carried out in anesthetized animals by Per Andersen, professor of neurophysiology at the University of Oslo, in the 1960s. Andersen and his associates were largely responsible for working out the neurophysiological properties of the three-stage hippocampal circuit. Basic to the study of the neurophysiology of the hippocampus is an understanding of its neuroanatomy, a task begun by Ramon y Cajal and continued to the present day by neuroanatomists using increasingly more powerful methods. Knowledge gained in this prior research made my experiment possible.

*200   It is possible by pharmacological means to deplete a rat's hippocampus selectively of norepinephrine. The animal may then be tested for neuronal gating effects in experiments of the type described. By studying the gating at the first stage of the three-stage chain, it has been determined that depleting norepinephrine eliminates the gating effect. See D. Dahl, W. H. Bailey, and J. Winson, "Effect of Norepinephrine Depletion of Hippocampus on Neuronal Transmission from Perforant Pathway Through Dentate Gyrus," *Journal of Neurophysiology*, 1983, Vol. 49, p. 123. Further studies are being performed to delineate the neural mechanisms that are operative. Based on known characteristics of norepinephrine, a modulatory action on the ability of incoming signals to fire hippocampal neurons might be expected. Other inputs from the brain stem have also been found that influence neuronal transmission. There are apparently complicated brain-stem systems which at least in part control the gating phenomenon.

Chapter 9, Hypothesis

210   H. P. Roffwarg, J. H. Herman, C. Bowe-Anders, and E. S. Tauber, "The Effects of Sustained Alterations of Waking Visual Input on Dream Content," Chapter 9 in A. M. Arkis,

Page   J. S. Antrobus, and S. J. Ellman, eds., *The Mind in Sleep* (Hillsdale, N.J.: Lawrence Erlbaum Associates, 1978).

214   D. Foulkes, *Children's Dreams* (New York: John Wiley and Sons, 1972).

214   "There was a bunch . . ." ibid. p. 213.

215   "Both by the nature . . ." ibid. p. 214.

*220   In mammals, prefrontal cortex sends an important output projection to the basal ganglia, a subcortical group of nuclei mediating voluntary movements. In reptiles, where behavioral responses are largely determined by genetic mechanisms rather than by learning, there is no prefrontal (nor any other neocortex), and the basal ganglia play a major role in governing behavior. The prefrontal cortex does not simply take over the function of the basal ganglia in mammals. Rather, the basal ganglia are integrated into a system in which the prefrontal cortex exerts executive control.

During the ontogenetic development of a young animal, the course of evolution seems to be repeated. While the prefrontal cortex is forming its internal connections and is not yet fully operational, the basal ganglia exert control. Goldman-Rakic and her colleagues showed this, using tests in monkeys which sensitively measure prefrontal cortex function. (The tests involve the ability of a monkey to remember the spatial location of an object after a time delay.) The prefrontal cortex was made nonfunctional in a reversible manner by cooling it locally with implanted probes. This was done in monkeys ranging in age from nine months to three years. The effect of prefrontal cooling was minimal in the youngest animals—they could perform the task. Presumably other brain regions were in charge. Cooling had more and more of a deleterious effect as the monkeys grew older; in the older animals the prefrontal cortex was the brain structure governing the task. A further study by the same investigators suggested that the governing structure in younger animals was probably the group of basal ganglia, for destroying part of this group impaired performance on the task while cooling (or destroying) the prefrontal cortex in monkeys of this age had not. For a comprehensive review of brain development including that of prefrontal cortex see P. S. Goldman, "Maturation of the Mammalian Ner-

Page

vous System and the Ontogeny of Behavior" in J. S. Rosen-
blatt, Robert A. Hende, Evelyn Shaw, and Colin Beer, eds.,
Advances in the Study of Behavior (New York: Academic
Press, 1976), Vol. 7.

221   Rosalind D. Cartwright, *Night Life, Explorations in Dreaming*
(Englewood Cliffs, N.J.: Prentice-Hall, 1977), p. 24. Cartwright recounts several interesting series of dreams obtained in
the sleep laboratory as well as a commentary on the psychology of dreaming.

223   "We started back . . ." ibid., p. 27.

225   "But it was not only his . . ." see p. 125.

225   R. Greenberg and C. Pearlman, "If Freud Only Knew: A Re-
consideration of Psychoanalytic Dream Theory," *International
Review of Psycho-analysis*, 1978, Vol. 5, p. 71.

*227   Further light was shed on the actual incidents surrounding the
Irma dream by Frank R. Hartman, "A Reappraisal of Emma
Episode and the Specimen Dream," *Journal of the American
Psychoanalytic Association*, July 1983, Vol. 31, p. 555. The
unpublished diaries of Princess Marie Bonaparte made available to Hartman reveal the possibility that the Irma to whom
Freud referred when he recounted Oskar Rie's report that
"She is better, but not quite well" was not Emma (Eckstein),
his patient who had been operated on by Fliess, but a second
patient Freud was treating for hysteria at the time, Anna
Hammerschlag Lichtheim. Rie was close to Anna's family and
might well have visited Anna before coming to see Freud on
the day before the Irma dream. In addition Freud makes a
comment in *The Interpretation of Dreams* that points toward
Anna as the Irma of his dream. He notes that in real life
Irma's family name bore a remarkable similarity to the liqueur
Ananas that Rie brought as a gift. If we suppose that Freud
stated that the similarity was to Anna's family name rather
than to her given name in order to disguise her identity, then
the patient Freud referred to in his comments on the Irma
dream may well have been Anna Hammerschlag Lichtheim.

Assuming then that Freud treated two patients, Emma who
had been operated on by Fliess several months prior to the
Irma dream and Anna whose case, following Oskar Rie's report, was the immediate subject of Freud's concern, what was

Page the unconscious message conveyed by the Irma dream? I suggest that it was very much the same as I have previously stated, namely: My patient (Anna) is in trouble as I am in my treatment of her. How can she be helped? Breuer's cathartic method will cure her, and I will be saved.

The line of association is the following. Anna worries Freud. She is resisting his analytic suggestions and remains ill with severe hysterical symptoms. Freud feels inadequate in his treatment. He in fact writes a report to Breuer to justify himself. In the dream Freud's unconscious thoughts immediately revert back to the traumatic and very similar situation concerning Emma. Here Freud was inadequate again; by referring Emma to Fliess he was almost responsible for her demise. The two patients are consolidated in the dream. The dramatic operation on Emma forms the main narrative, and blame is placed squarely on Fliess. But Rie, who was the bearer of bad tidings with regard to Anna, becomes the culprit in the dream. The two men are similar, both are facile but not thorough, and they are not to be trusted. The main message remains: My patient and I will be rescued by Breuer's cathartic method.

It should be noted that Hartman, in agreement with Alan C. Elms, interprets the Irma dream as referring to Freud's concerns over impregnating his wife Martha. Martha was six months pregnant at the time of the dream. The reader may wish to refer to Alan C. Elms, "Freud, Irma, Martha: Sex and Marriage in the Dream of Irma Injection," *Psychoanalytic Review*, 1980, Vol. 67, p. 83, for this interpretation and a summary of several others.

A definitive interpretation of the Irma dream will never be achieved. Freud clearly fell short in what he published; his omission of negative associations to Fliess can hardly be construed otherwise. A complete understanding would have required Freud being analyzed by someone else and exhaustively working his way through the many lines of association present in the dream. The interpretation I have presented is based on two clues. One is the formation of the dream narrative to serve the "need for representability." The reader will recall Freud's example of a dream in which a deluge of rain was arranged to represent the concept of "superfluous." Dreams are not constructed for purpose of representability lightly; when a concept is so portrayed, there is usually an essential message to be decoded. In the Irma dream, Breuer's statement about dysentery appears to be an example of the dream narrative turned to the purpose of representability. What better way to make the point? Irma's illness is at once a re-creation of the Fliess incident weighing so heavily on Freud's mind (with Fliess's blame repressed) and a physical illness about which Breuer's statement can be made. The statement itself claiming that dysentery will follow and the patient will recover strikes one as having no purpose other than to represent psychoanalysis, the outgrowth of the cathartic method, and what it will accomplish. (Freud called the statement foolish, designed to deride Breuer.) And the fact that Breuer, father of the method, makes the pronouncement completes the message perfectly. The second clue has to do with Freud's state of mind at the time of the Irma dream. He was much concerned with the adequacy of his treatment. Rescue from this insecurity by the fatherlike figure Breuer, whose method was indeed capable of accomplishing this feat, was an appropriate unconscious thought under the circumstances. True or not, this interpretation serves to illustrate both the kind of concept—rescue by a father—which may remain part of the adult unconscious and the flow of unconscious thought in reaction to important daily events that may be expressed by dreams.

228   "The dream gives a true picture . . ." C. G. Jung, *Modern Man in Search of a Soul* (New York: Harcourt, Brace and World, 1933), p. 4.

*231   For a discussion of the issue of children's laboratory dreams versus dreams at home in which a child may be questioned by a parent or child psychiatrist (thus eliciting a transference reaction), the reader may want to refer to Steven L. Ablon and John E. Mack, "Children's Dreams Reconsidered," in Albert J. Solnit, Ruth S. Eissler, Anna Freud, Marianne Kris, and Peter B. Neubauer, eds., *The Psychoanalytic Study of the Child* (New Haven, Conn.: Yale University Press, 1980), p. 179.

232   See *The Question of Animal Awareness* by Donald R. Griffin (New York: The Rockefeller University Press, 1976).

Page   *232 Eccles's thesis may be found in Karl Popper and John C. Eccles, *The Self and Its Brain* (Berlin: Springer International, 1977). Sperry's viewpoint is given in "Mind-Brain Interactions: Mentalism, Yes; Dualism, No," *Neuroscience*, 1980, Vol. 5, p. 195. The mind-brain problem is discussed extensively in the above two works. For initial reading on this subject I recommend Douglas R. Hofstadter and Daniel C. Dennett, *The Mind's I* (New York: Basic Books, 1981).

     *234 In Freud's theoretical framework, repression is a mechanism operating in the unconscious. Just as an unconscious censor prevents destructive instinctual urges from breaking through in dreams, so in the waking state, censorship exerted by the unconscious part of the ego represses such urges and prevents them from reaching consciousness. Thus, "The ego notices that the satisfaction of an emerging instinctual demand would conjure up one of the well remembered situations of danger." (An example would be a boy's Oedipal wish to kill his father with the consequent unconsciously perceived danger—that is, castration.)

Freud goes on to say that this leads to the generation of unconscious anxiety, which activates an unconscious part of the ego. Then, "This instinctual cathexis must therefore be suppressed, stopped, made powerless. . . . The ego . . . now carries out the repression of the dangerous instinctive impulse. . . . [This must] be in fact a process that is neither conscious nor preconscious, but taking place between quotas of energy in some unimaginable substratum." *Standard Edition*, Vol. XXII, p. 89.

The phenomenon of resistance in psychoanalysis is explained in a similar fashion. During the course of the analysis, repressed unconscious ideas begin to be brought to consciousness. Anxiety develops, and repression now takes the form of resistance, the denial of what is emerging or an unwillingness to continue the psychoanalytic process. The analyst must work carefully to overcome this resistance. If the unconscious material can be made conscious, particularly by interpretation of dreams and the transference relationship, its irrationality exposed, the patient's self-destructive behavior or symptoms will, it is hoped, be dissipated.

The hypothesis presented here differs in the following respect. It is not the case that a continuous dynamic process occurs, in which emerging instinctual urges provoke anxiety and are then repressed. Rather, the mechanisms Freud observed and called unconscious are part of an individual's strategy of thought and behavior laid down early in life. Anxiety and repression do take place, when for example the analyst and patient manage to come to grips with an unconscious thought like the Oedipal wish. But the repression is a conscious or preconscious reaction to a painful thought, akin to the repression of a memory of a war trauma. The present hypothesis suggests the source of the difficulty in producing behavioral change once an unconscious idea is brought to light. Although insight is achieved, and the patient may understand and decry the painful flaw in his or her psychological makeup, the patient may not be able to change it or may only be able to change it with great difficulty, for the flaw is part of an unconscious strategy set down during the critical period of brain development.

*234 Libet's experiments are reported in B. Libet, E. W. Wright, Jr., B. Feinstein, and D. K. Pearl, "Subjective Referral of the Timing for a Conscious Sensory Experience," *Brain*, 1979, Vol. 102, p. 193. The following is a more complete description of the studies.

The diagnosis and treatment of the patients Libet used in his studies required that electrodes be inserted into their brains. This was carried out by a neurosurgeon, Bertram Feinstein, while the patients were awake so that they could respond to questions during the diagnostic procedure. (As I have mentioned, the brain has no pain receptors, and so the patients felt no discomfort.) In many patients the electrodes remained in place for a week or more to judge the course of therapy, and these patients could be studied outside the operating room under ambulatory conditions. During the diagnostic procedure and afterward, Libet was able to use the implanted electrodes to test the touch system of the brain to investigate consciousness. A mild electric stimulus was applied to the skin of one hand. It is known that this stimulation—indeed any skin stimulus—is translated at the skin into a neural signal that passes through one relay in the brain stem, a second in the thalamus, and then arrives at the portion of the neocortex specialized for touch (somatosensory cortex). Using a recording electrode in neocortex, Libet could measure the incoming signal. Signal transmission time from the hand was very short, about 15 thousandths of a second, and the patient reported that he felt a tingling sensation of his skin at that time. The measurement of conduction time from the skin of the hand to neocortex had been made many times before in monkeys, and what Libet found was unexceptional.

Libet now considered the question of consciousness. To the area of sensory neocortex from which he had just taken recordings, Libet now applied a mild, electrical stimulus. The patient reported a tingling sensation on the skin of the hand although the skin itself was not stimulated. This too was not surprising. Had the hand received a stimulus, the neural signal would have arrived at the neocortex, and stimulating the neocortex directly merely mimicked the natural neural signal. The patient could distinguish between the stimulus applied to the hand and that applied to the neocortex—the tingling produced by stimulating the neocortex seemed to come from a different part of the hand than the directly applied skin stimulus, and the sensations themselves were somewhat different. Stimuli were now applied to the hand and the neocortex simultaneously. One would expect that the patient would feel the two tingling sensations at about the same time. But this was not the case. Instead, the sensation caused by stimulating the neocortex was felt considerably later than the tingling produced by the stimulus applied to the skin. To determine the extent of this time lag, Libet stimulated the neocortex first and, about one quarter second later, stimulated the skin. The actual skin stimulation, though applied one quarter of a second later, was still the first to be perceived. Only when the neocortex was stimulated about one-half second before the skin did the patient feel that the two sensations were occurring simultaneously. Thus when the skin stimulus was applied, the patient felt the sensation in a very short time, at virtually the same time that the neural signal arrived at the neocortex.

But when the neocortex was stimulated directly, the sensation was not felt for one-half second.

It is only logical to assume that the brain process whereby the sensation became conscious takes time. The one-half second between stimulation of the neocortex and the patient feeling the tingling sensation is a reasonable length of time for the brain to carry out the process. But then some mechanism must intervene when the touch signal is real, when it originates in the hand and proceeds through two relay points before reaching neocortex, to make it appear to the conscious mind that the sensation is felt at the time the signal reaches the neocortex, rather than one-half second later when it actually does become conscious.

Libet performed further experiments of the type described here to determine the point in the neural circuit at which this mechanism intervenes. He reasoned that it was somewhere before the signal reached the neocortex, for when the neocortex was stimulated directly, it took one-half second for the sensation to become effective for perception. His experiments localized the site of action. When the normal signal passes the last relay of the circuit in the thalamus, it appears that a process is initiated which corrects subjective awareness by the amount of time required for conscious perception to occur. In commenting on the results of his experiments, Libet noted that the one-half second required for a sensation to become conscious, allowed time for repression to occur.

One may ask how those postulating a nonneural basis for consciousness explained Libet's findings. Sir John Eccles, in discussing the experiments, believes that it is exactly at the point where the time required for processing sensation into consciousness is eliminated, so as to bring sensation into time synchrony with its conscious perception, that a nonneural or spiritual entity intervenes to accomplish the task. Others, believing in a nonneural basis for consciousness, suggest that consciousness is not necessarily spiritual in origin but nevertheless is derived from a separate, nonneural entity.

*235   It may be appropriate at this point to relate the content of this book to other terms that have been used to describe the human mind. I see three realms of the mind. First, there is consciousness, the immediate, undeniable "I" in each of us that perceives, thinks, feels, and acts. This is the last frontier of neuroscience, probably the most difficult realm of the mind to explain on the basis of brain function, if indeed it is based in the brain. (Most neuroscientists believe that it is, and Libet's approach may provide a path for investigation.) Second, there is the realm of feeling, motivation, and strategies of behavior, operating on levels that are beneath conscious awareness—the "Psyche" with its roots in the unconscious. How this is derived from the brain is the subject of my hypothesis. Third, there is the cognitive mind, the realm of Hippocrates' "wisdom and knowledge," the analysis of sensory events and objects of the outside world, memory, reasoning, and learning. I have also described areas of brain function that underlie cognitive function such as memory; these functions constitute the raw material for the psyche as well as for growth of knowledge. The cognitive mind had its own major figure, its own Freud in the person of psychologist Jean Piaget. Neuroscience has as its ultimate goal the understanding of all the aspects of mind and their relationships to the brain. The mysteries of the psyche and cognition are slowly being unraveled with consciousness a more distant target.

*235   However, a few such cases continue to turn up in neurological practice. These patients may exhibit paralysis, loss of sensation, or partial blindness following an accident or associated with a fear of a disabling or life-threatening disease. There is no discernible neurological basis for the symptoms. They may disappear spontaneously or be relieved by treatment which is purely psychological in content. They may also persist for long periods of time. A present-day evaluation of hysteria may be found in E. Slater and M. Roth, *Clinical Psychiatry*, 3d edition (Baltimore: Williams and Wilkins, 1969), p. 103. To the reader interested in hysteria I also recommend D. W. Abse, *The Diagnosis of Hysteria* (Bristol: John Wright and Sons Ltd.; London: Simkin Marshall Ltd., 1950). This is a study of British and Indian soldiers referred for psychiatric evaluation during the Second World War. Abse reports the differential diagnosis and treatment of a number of cases of hysteria which developed under the stress of war. In these, the classical hysterical symptoms appeared, including hysterical epileptic fits. Abse notes that hysteria was much more prevalent among the Indian soldiers than among the British (of 644 Indian psychiatric admissions, 370 were diagnosed as hysterics while of 669 British admissions, 161 were hysterics). He attributes this greater tendency of Indian soldiers to develop hysteria to their relative psychological immaturity as compared to their British counterparts, a view consistent with earlier findings of Briquet who compared hysteria in country and city girls (see Chapter 3, p. 73). The historical decline of hysteria may in some way be related to the growing sophistication of the general populace.

235   Kubie on multiple personality: L. S. Kubie, "Some Unsolved Problems of Psychoanalytic Psychotherapy," in F. Fromm-Reichman and J. L. Moreno, eds., *Progress in Psychotherapy* (New York: Grune and Stratton, 1956).

236   Kubie's view of hypnosis is given in L. S. Kubie, "Hypnotism," *Archives of General Psychiatry*, 1961, Vol. 4, p. 66.

236   Hilgard's work is described in "Divided Consciousness in Hypnosis: The Implications of the Hidden Observer," Chapter 3 in E. Fromm and R. E. Shor, eds., *Hypnosis* (New York: Aldine Publishing Co., 1979).

236   Soldier hypnotized to earlier life stages: E. R. Hilgard, L. S. Kubie, and E. Pumpian-Mindlin, eds., *Psychoanalysis as a Science* (Stanford, Calif.: Stanford University Press, 1952), p. 55.

237   "In every case we are . . ." E. Bleuler, *Dementia Praecox or the Group of Schizophrenias* (New York: International Universities Press, 1950), p. 9.

238   "The real trouble begins . . ." C. G. Jung, *The Psychology of Dementia Praecox*, Bollingen Series XX (Princeton, N.J.: Princeton University Press, 1974), p. 162.

238   Genetic transmission in schizophrenia: S. S. Kety, D. Rosenthal, P. H. Wender, F. Schulsinger, and B. Jacobsen, "Mental Illness in the Biological and Adoptive Families of Adopted Individuals Who Have Become Schizophrenic," in R. Fieve, D. Rosenthal, and H. Brill, eds., *Genetic Research in Psychiatry* (Baltimore: Johns Hopkins University Press, 1975), p. 147.

238   Blood flow studies in the neocortex: D. H. Ingvar, "Hyperfrontal Distribution of the Cerebral Grey Matter Flow in

Page   Resting Wakefulness; on the Functional Anatomy of the Conscious State," *Acta Neurologica Scandinavia*, 1969, Vol. 60, p. 12.

239   "The high frontal activity . . ." ibid., p. 12.

239   Norepinephrine in visual cortex: T. Kasamatsu and J. D. Pettigrew, "Preservation of Binocularity after Monocular Deprivation in the Striate Cortex of Kittens Treated with 6-Hydroxydopamine," *Journal of Comparative Neurology*, 1979, Vol. 185, p. 139.

Chapter 10, Epilogue

*241   The theory was evolved over a period of years as an explanatory framework for my own and others' research findings. I first presented my ideas on the evolutionary basis of dreaming and the story of the echidna at Symposium on Brain Function and Behavior held by the Harry F. Guggenheim Foundation at Millbrook, New York, in 1976, referred to in Robin Fox, *The Red Lamp of Incest* (E. P. Dutton, N.Y., 1980), p. 177, and in comments at a symposium on the functions of sleep sponsored by the City University of New York in 1980, cited in Ernest Hartmann, "The Functions of Sleep and Memory Processing" in W. Fishbein, ed. *Sleep Dreams in Memory* (New York: SP Medical and Scientific Books, 1981), p. 111.

244   "The active contents of the unconscious . . ." C. G. Jung, *Modern Man in Search of a Soul* (New York: Harcourt, Brace and Co., 1934), p. 90.

244   "I suggest that there is . . ." Robert J. Stoller, *Sexual Excitement, Dynamics of Erotic Life* (New York: Pantheon, 1979), p. 207.

*244   This might be one step in the strategy of obtaining psychoanalytic data to be compared with the findings of neuroscience as they are developed in the areas of memory and information processing during sleep.

Glossary

Action potential. Electrical pulse generated at the body of the neuron and transmitted out along the axon. The action potential is the means by which one neuron signals information to another.

Alpha rhythm. A 10 per second rhythmic electrical potential recorded in the neocortical EEG during resting with the eyes closed. Although the source of alpha rhythm is presumed to be generated in the visual cortex, its source has not yet been accurately determined. The function of the rhythm is unknown.

Amygdala. A structure of the limbic system lying beneath the temporal lobes associated with affect and memory.

Anterior thalamic nuclei. Nuclei (anatomically distinct clusters of neurons) in the forward part of the thalamus that constitutes part of the limbic system. The function of these cell groups is not known, but they provide an anatomical link between the limbic system and the neocortex.

Axon. The output fibers of a neuron along which the action potential is transmitted.

Basal ganglia. Structures in the forebrain associated with the initiation of movement. The basal ganglia receive an important input from the prefrontal cortex, which presumably acts as the executive control in the choice of behavior. In submammalian species, there is no prefrontal cortex and the basal ganglia constitute the entire forebrain component of the movement-related neural system.

Brain stem. The stalk or base of the brain, responsible for basic life-sustaining functions such as respiration, and involved in both sensory and motor function. The brain stem (inherited from reptilian species) has been integrated into the mammalian brain by the formation of extensive connections with the forebrain. The sources of both REM sleep and theta rhythm lie in the brain stem as do the norepinephrine containing neurons that send axons to the hippocampus and neocortex.

Cerebellum. Structure lying atop the upper part of the brain stem forming a part of the brain system controlling movement. Its precise function is not known, but it is thought to be involved with the coordination or memory of movements.

Cerebral cortex. See neocortex.

Cingulate cortex. Strip of neocortex lying near the midline of the brain—a part of the limbic system.

Cortical column. A vertical array of interconnected neurons of the neocortex, forming a column oriented perpendicular to the surface of the brain which constitutes a processing unit or module. A cortical column contains on the order of 100 neurons. The neocortex is believed to consist of some 600 million of such columns engaged in sensory, movement-related, and associative tasks.

Critical period. A well-defined period of time during the early stages of brain development in which experience guides anatomical or functional connectivity. Such connectivity may then be difficult or impossible to change later in life.

Dendrite. The input fibers of a neuron. Incoming signals to a target neuron act on the neuron's dendrites. Each neuron is an integrating unit, acting according to its own inherent logic to fire action potentials or not in response to inputs to its dendrites and cell body.

Dopamine. One of the three monoamine neurotransmitters. Several lines of evidence have linked malfunction of the dopamine system of the brain with both schizophrenia and Parkinson's syndrome.

EEG. Electroencephalogram, the electrical potential generated by the neurons of the neocortex, measured by electrodes placed over the skull. Discovered by Hans Berger in the early 1930s, this indicator of neocortical function has been used extensively in sleep research as well as in the diagnosis of neurological disease.

Electrode. A sensing element, usually a fine wire, a fine glass tube filled with a conducting fluid, or a metal disk, used to record electrical signals of the brain. Electrodes are also used to stimulate nerve cells or fibers.

Entorhinal cortex. An area of neocortex that receives highly processed information relating to all sensory modalities from other areas of neocortex and the limbic system. The major input to the hippocampus originates in the entorhinal cortex and is transmitted to it by the perforant pathway.

Ganglion cells. Neurons within the retina whose output fibers (axons) constitute the optic nerve projecting to the lateral geniculate nucleus of the thalamus.

Gate. See neural gate.

Hippocampus. A major structure of the limbic system serving as the gateway for the transmission of information from the entorhinal cortex to other limbic system components. The hippocampus is intimately associated with memory.

Inferotemporal cortex. Lower portion of the temporal lobes in which it is believed that visual information, after sequential processing steps in other visually related areas, is analyzed to distinguish among specific objects.

Lamella. The processing module of the hippocampus. A thin cross-sectional slice of the hippocampus that contains its basic three-stage circuit.

Lateral geniculate. Nucleus of cells in the thalamus that serves as the visual relay station between the eye and the primary visual cortex.

Limbic system. A series of interconnected structures in the forebrain, including the hippocampus and the amygdala, that is believed to serve as a central processing unit of the brain. The limbic system is involved in the processing of memory and in emotion. It is also closely associated anatomically with the prefrontal cortex, and thus presumably plays a role in the determination of behavior. The precise function of the limbic system is unknown.

Mammillary bodies. A component of the limbic system. A limbic system circuit connects the hippocampus to the mammillary bodies, which in turn send axons to the anterior thalamic nuclei.

Mediodorsal nucleus. The thalamic relay for the prefrontal cortex. Among other inputs, the mediodorsal nucleus receives an input from the amygdala, thus providing a limbic system input to the prefrontal cortex.

Medulla. The lower part of the brain stem.

Monoamines. These are norepinephrine, dopamine, and serotonin, all neurotransmitters believed to act as modulators in the brain. Several lines of evidence have implicated the monoamines in mental disorders.

Motor cortex. Part of neocortex associated with movement.

Neocortex. The sheet of neural tissue about 1/10 inch thick, that covers the brain. The neocortex consists of approximately 50 billion neurons arranged in functional columns. The most significant change that occurred in the structure of the brain during the course of evolution was the expansion of the neocortex. In higher animals and in man, the expansion of the neocortex within the limited confines of the skull, caused the neocortical sheet to fold upon itself in accordionlike fashion to form convolutions. It is believed to be the site of the highest level of sensory and mental functions.

Neuron. A cell of the nervous system specialized for the processing and the transmission of information. The neuron consists of dendrites on which inputs are received, a cell body, and an axon, which transmits the action potential or output signal of the cell to other neurons. Axons may branch along their course, and thus a single neuron may transmit information to many others.

Neuronal gating. A phenomenon in the brain in which passage of a signal through one or more neurons that form a junction of a circuit may or may not be restricted (gate closed or open). Neuronal gating occurs in the hippocampus at each junction of the basic three stage circuit within the lamella, the gates being open or closed depending on the behavioral state of the animal.

Neurotransmitter. The chemical substance released from the synapse at the far end of the axon by the action potential. The neurotransmitter acts on a dendrite or the cell body of the target neuron to excite or inhibit it.

Norepinephrine. A monoamine neurotransmitter. Norepinephrine neurons of locus coeruleus send axons to both neocortex and hippocampus. These cells fire at their maximum rate when an animal is brought to an alert state. This is believed to increase the efficiency of processing sensory information in the neocortex and to affect neuronal gating in the hippocampus.

Off-line processing. In computer science, the acquisition of input information and its temporary storage in computer memory until a time when processing components are available.

Perforant pathway. Axons connecting the entorhinal cortex to the first stage of the hippocampal three-stage circuit.

Phoneme. An elemental speech sound.

Prefrontal cortex. The forwardmost area of the neocortex, believed to be the region that governs strategies for behavior.

Primary visual cortex. The first neocortical region to receive and analyze visual information.

REM sleep. Rapid eye movement sleep. It is the sleep stage characterized by rapid movement of the eyes under closed lids, irregular breathing, and other physiological indicators. Dreaming occurs during REM sleep.

Septum. Component of the limbic system with extensive connections to hippocampus and other limbic structures. Neurons in the medial part of the septum act as pacemaker cells for hippocampal theta rhythm.

Serotonin. A monoamine transmitter. Its function is unknown.

Slow-wave sleep. In animals, the stages of sleep characterized by large slow-waves in the neocortical EEG. Slow-wave and REM sleep alternate during the course of a sleep episode. Slow-wave sleep in animals corresponds to sleep stages 2, 3, and 4 in man.

Striate cortex. Primary visual cortex.

Synapse. The expansion of the axon at its far end from which neurotransmitter is released by an arriving action potential, thus passing information to another neuron.

Temporal lobe. The region of the neocortex that lies beneath the temples. It includes the inferotemporal cortex that mediates advanced stages of visual processing.

Thalamus. A structure lying beneath the neocortex, in which groups of neurons act as relay stations in the transmission of information to the neocortex. There are also reciprocal connections from neocortex to the thalamic relays. The precise action of the relay neurons is one area of current neuroscientific study.

Theta rhythm. An approximately 6 per second rhythm generated in particular groups of neurons of the hippocampus and entorhinal cortex. In lower animals the rhythm occurs during species-specific waking states as well as during REM sleep.

Index

Page numbers in *italics* indicate illustrations or captions.

Abandonment, fear of, 149, 246
Abraham, Karl, 130, 132
Abreaction, 262n.
Abse, D. W., 279n.–80n.
Abstract ideas, 112
    and brain mechanisms for
        unconscious integration, 217–18
Abzug, Charles, 196
Adaptation, 139, 155, 225
Adler, Alfred, 129, 138–39, 140,
    144, 145, 146, 149, 150, 153
Adrian, Edgar, 38
Aetiology of Hysteria, The, 81, 87
Aggression, 135, 230–31, 246
Agoraphobia, 113, 115
Albert Einstein College of
    Medicine, 210
Alcohol addiction, 157
Allison, Truett, 53–55, 185
Alpha rhythm, 38–39, 42, *44*, 181,
    186–87
American Psychiatric Association,
    157
American Psychoanalytic
    Association, 147, 157
Amnesia, 12–17, 233
    and electroconvulsive therapy,
        250n.
    and hypnosis, 79

Amygdala, 30, *199*, 242, 253n.,
    267n.
    and emotion, 31–32
    location of, *28, 32–33*
    removal of, 11, 13–14, 28
    and sensory perception, 28–29
Anal stage, 134
"Analysis Terminable and
    Interminable," 158
Andersen, Per, 270n.
Animal magnetism, 76–77
Anna O., 67–71, 74, 78, 81, 86, 87,
    88
Anorexia nervosa, 235
Anterior thalamic nuclei, 30–31, *32–
    33*
Antidepressant drugs, 194, 195
Antipsychotic drugs, 195
Anti-Semitism, 132
Archetypes, 145, 146
Arduini, Arnaldo, 180–82
Arousal state
    and hippocampal theta rhythm,
        181–83
    and neural processing in
        hippocampus, 197–98, 200–2
    and norepinephrine actions, 193,
        196
    See also Sleep
Aserinsky, Eugene, 40–42

Association cortex, 178, 185, 219
and REM sleep, 46
Astigmatism, 173, 174
Audition. *See* Hearing
Autosuggestion, 72, 77
Axons, *22*, 219
growth of, 163, *164, 165*
and the monoamine system, 192–93

Basal ganglia, 58, 189, 205, 220, 271n.
Basel University, 130
Beauchamp, Christine, 75–76, 88, 147
Behavior
critical period for organization of, 163, 174–79
and limbic system functions, 29, 31–34
and neural processing in hippocampus, 196
and prefrontal cortex, 58–59, 205–6
See also Species-specific behaviors
Behavior modification, 157
Bekhterev, V. M., 59
Berger, Hans, 37–38, 181
Berger rhythm, 38
Bernays, Martha, 65, 66, 86, 128, 273n.
Bernheim, Hippolyte, 77, 79, 80
Bettelheim, Bruno, 159
"Beyond the Pleasure Principle," 134
Binocular vision, 173
Biological clock, 36
Blakemore, Colin, 172–73, 174
Bleuler, Eugen, 131, 132, 137, 237
Blood pressure, 35–36
Bloom, Floyd, 193
Boas, Franz, 133
Body movement, 189
Body temperature, 35–36, 55
Braid, James, 77

Brain development, 162–79
Brain stem, 30, 32–33, 243
and hippocampal theta rhythm generation, 189
and movement inhibition in REM sleep, 46–47
and neural processing in hippocampus, 192, 193, 201, 270n.
and sleep cycle control, 50
Brain weight, 162–63
Breuer, Josef, 3, 67–71, 78, 79, 80, 81, 82, 86, 88–89, 94, 96, 98, 100, 109, 110, 118, 131, 133, 150, 217, 226, 227, 273n.–74n.
Brill, Abraham, 61, 130, 133, 147
Briquet, Dr., 73–74
British Medical Journal, 9, 161
Broca, Pierre-Paul, 2, 29–30
Brücke, Ernst, 63, 64, 65, 66, 67, 86
Bucy, Paul, 32
Burghölzli Psychiatric Hospital, 130–31, 137, 147, 237
Butyrophenones, 195

California Institute of Technology, 239
Cartwright, Rosalind, 221–24, 229
Castration fear, 117
Cat Behavior, 174
Categorical perception, 166–69
Cathartic method, 70, 71, 75, 78, 79, 226, 227, 228, 273n.–74n.
Cell bodies, 19–*20*, 21, *22*
Cerebellum, *32–33*, 189
Cerebral blood flow, 238–39
Charcot, Jean-Martin, 66, 67, 71–74, 77–79, 235
Children's dreams, 214, 229–32, 243–44
Chlorpromazine, 195
Cingulate cortex, 30–31, *32–33*
Circadian variations of physiological function, 35–37
Clark, Ronald W., 86

Clark University, 132
Cocaine, 96, 97
Cognitive mind, 279n.
Collective unconscious, 145, 146
Color perception, 24, 26
Columbia University, 51, 266n.
Columbia University School of
    Psychoanalysis, 129
Compulsion to repetition, 134–35
Condensation, 108–10, 114, 151,
    214, 217
Consciousness, *116*, 232–35, 247
    neural basis for, 277n.–78n., 279n.
Cooper, Grahame, 172–73
Corpus callosum, *32–33*
Cortical column, 26–27, 169, 201,
    252n.
    neuroanatomy of, 185
Critical period, 7, 209, 239, 246
    in audition, 162–63, 166–69, 178–
    79
    impressions processed into
        unconscious during, 220–21
    in predation in cats, 162, 174–79
    in vision, 162, 169–74, 178–79
Critique of Psychoanalysis, 203
Croonian Lectures, 161
Curare, 181, 187, 188

Darwin, Charles, 62, 63
Day residue, 101, 119, 211, 219,
    222, 226
Death instinct, 135, 137, 152
Defense theory, 84, 87, 137, 214,
    215, 216, 262n.
Delta waves, 42, *44*
Dement, William, 42–44, 47–49, 51
*Dementia Praecox or the Group of
    Schizophrenias*, 131
Dendrites, 19–*20*, 21, *22*, 219
    growth of, 163, *164*, *165*
Dependency, 77, 79
Depression, 156
    electroconvulsive therapy for, 14–
    15

and the monoamines, 194
and physical brain function, 34,
    194, 236–37
Depth perception, 24, 26, 169, 170,
    174
Developmental explanation of
    mental organization, 115
Despine, Dr., 75, 77
Displacement, 108, 111, 114, 151,
    214, 219, 233–34
Dissociation, 87
Don's dreams, 221–23, 229
Dopamine, 192–93, 195
    and schizophrenia, 238–40
Downstate Medical Center, 188
Dream distortion, 108, 114–15, *116*,
    151, 155, 160, 210, 214, 215,
    230
Dreams, 5–7, 154, 158, 241, 245
    Adler's view of, 139
    biology of, 34–60
    brain mechanisms underlying,
        214–19
    content of, *116*, 243–44
    evolution of, 191, 204, 209–10
    Freud's view of, 3–4, 91–126,
        148–49, 151–52
    and information processing, 210–
    12
    Jung's view of, 145–46, 228
    meaning of, 191, 221–32
    and transference, 135
    and traumatic neuroses, 134–35,
    147
    See also Children's dreams;
        Dream distortion; Irma dream,
        Freud's; Symbolism in dreams;
        Wish fulfillment theory
Drug addiction, 157
Drugs, psychoactive, 157, 193–95,
    235
    and neurotransmitter actions, 21
Dual personality. *See* Multiple
    personality
Duck-billed platypus, 53, 242

Early experience, *116*, 160, 179, 220–21
Eccles, John, 232, 278n.
Echidna (spiny anteater), 53–*54*, 55–*57*, 58–59, 185, 193, 204, 208, 243
Ego, 103, 135–37, 150, 152, 153
Ego and the Id, The, 135
Ego psychology, 117, 137, 139, 150
Eichenbaum, Howard, 268n.
Electra complex, 105–6, 153
Electroconvulsive therapy, 14–16, 250n.
Electroencephalogram (EEG), 78, 181, 186–87, 221
  and sleep study, 35, 37, 39–42, 44, 46, 48, 54–55
Electrotherapy, 78
Ellenberger, Henri, 71, 74, 79
Elms, Alan, 273n.
Emily's dreams, 214, 230
Emma, 94–95, 102, 119–25, 225, 226, 227, 233, 272n.–73n.
Emotion, 220, 245
  brain mechanisms underlying, 29, 31–34
  within dreams, 230
Entorhinal cortex, 29, 180, 186, 189, 190, 191, 208
  and neural processing in hippocampus, 196–97, *198, 199*
Environment, 189, 190, 247
  and brain development in critical period, 172–73, 174, 178
  and learning, 205
  social, 235, 246–47
Epilepsy, 2, 10–11, 71, 200
  hysterical, 74, 77–78, 280n.
Erb, Wilhelm Heinrich, 78
Erikson, Erik, 101–2, 108, 150, 217
Eros, 135
Estelle, 75, 77
Evolution, 185, 189, 241, 245, 271n.
  and information processing during REM sleep, 206–12
Experience, 205, 214, 235

and learning, 176, 177, 178, 179
  See also Early experience
Exploration, 179, 184, 207

Fantasies, 89–90, 93, 106, 144, 230
Feature detection, 170, 173, 174, 185, 215, 241
Feinstein, Bertram, 276n.
Ferenczi, Sandor, 130, 133
Five Lectures on Psychoanalysis, 133
Fleischl, Ernst von, 96
Fliess, Wilhelm, 86, 99, 118–25, 128, 225–28, 233, 272n.–74n.
Foramen of Monro, 30
Fordham University, 142
Form detection, 24, 26
Fornix, *32–33*
Foulkes, David, 49, 214, 229–31, 244
Free association, 117, 138, 145, 148, 149, 150, 154, 156, 158, 159, 217, 243
  development of, 80–81
  and dream interpretation, 91–93, 102, 111, 113
  and unconscious associational network, 218–19
French Academy of Sciences, 77
Freud, Amalie (mother), 62–63
Freud, Anna (daughter), 119, 150
Freud, Anna (sister), 62–63
Freud, Jacob, 62–63
Freud, Martin, 107
Freud, Sigmund, 3–7, 34, 61, 210, 211, 214, 216, 217, 218, 219, 221, 231, 232, 233, 235, 241, 245, 263n., 275n., 276n.–77n.
  and Adler, 129, 138–39
  and the development of psychoanalysis, 127–51
  dream interpretation as developed by, 91–126
  early discoveries of, 62–90
  and Jung, 130–33, 137, 139–46
  scientific style of, 85–90

specimen dream of, 94–102, 108, 109, 110–11, 119, 124–25, 150, 217, 224–29, 231, 272n.–74n.
"Freud and the Soul," 159
Freudian slips, 128
Fromm, Eric, 150
Frontal lobotomy, 195
Fuster, Joaquim, 58, 205

Ganglion cells, 18–*19*
Genetic factors, 235, 238
   and critical period in brain development, 170, 173, 174, 178
   and hippocampal theta rhythm, 189
   See also Hereditary predisposition
Genital stage, 134
Gersuny, Dr., 119–21, 123–24
Glial cells, 163
Goldman-Rakic, Patricia, 220, 271n.
Graf, Max, 129
Green, John, 180–82, 187
Greenberg, Ramon, 225
Griffin, Donald, 232
Growth hormone, 56

Hall, Calvin, 216
Hall, G. Stanley, 132–33
Hallucination, 115
Haloperidol, 195
Hartford Hospital, 10
Hartman, Frank, R., 272n., 273n.
Hartmann, Ernest, 217
Hartmann, Heinz, 150
Harvard Medical School, 168
Harvard University, 22
Hearing, 18, *23–25*, 29
   columnar processing in, 27
   critical period in, 162–63, 166–69, 178–79
Heart rate, 35–36, 41
Hereditary predisposition, 72, 74, 144

See also Genetic factors
Hilgard, Ernest, 236
"Hippocampal Electrical Activity in Arousal," 182
Hippocampus, 5, 7, *32–33*, 58, 60
   function of, 201–2, 207, 241–42
   and H.M.'s syndrome, 11–17, 27–29
   and limbic system functions, 29–34
   and long-term memory, 15–17
   and memory consolidation, 212–13
   neuroanatomy of, 185–86, 196–97, *198, 199*
   neuronal gating in, 193–202, 208, 214, 237
   and sleep, 43–44, 180
   See also Theta rhythm, hippocampal
Hippocrates, 1, 2, 245, 279n.
Hirsch, Helmut, 173
H.M.'s syndrome, 10–17, 27–29, 180, 201, 207, 212, 250n., 252n.–53n.
Homosexuality, 117, 148–49, 155–56, 158, 222–23, 229
Hormones, 235
Horney, Karen, 150
Hubel, David, 22, 169, 170, 171
Hypersexuality, 32
Hypnogogic imagery, 210
Hypnoid states, 87
Hypnosis, 6, 72, 130
   and Anna O., 68–70
   Freud's use of, 79–80, 86
   history of, 73, 76–78
   and multiple personality, 235–36
Hysteria, 72, 125, 131, 134, 272n., 279n.–80n.
   and Anna O., 67–71
   Freud's theory of, 78–90, 92–93, 115, 117, 144, 152
   history of, 73–76
   incidence of, 149, 235, 280n.
Hysterical epilepsy, 74, 77–78, 280n.

Hysterical paralysis, 71, 72, 146, 279n.

Id, 103, 135–36, 150, 152, 154, 245, 246
Imprinting, 162
Inborn perceptual mechanism, 167
Infant sexuality theory, 151
  Adler's view of, 138–39, 152
  Freud's development of, 133–34, 152
  Jung's view of, 132, 139, 142–44, 146
  Krafft-Ebing's view of, 128
Inferiority complex, 138–39
Inferotemporal cortex, 24–25, 26, 28
Information processing, 32, 241
  and dreams, 210–12
  and hippocampal neural mechanisms, 197–202
  during REM sleep, 52–53, 206–12
  during slow-wave sleep, 208, 210
Information systems theory for psychoanalytic data, 155
Ingvar, David, 238–39
Instinct theory, 135
International Psychoanalytic Association, 129, 137, 139, 142, 146
Interneuronal connections, 163, 178
Interpretation of Dreams, The, 3, 6, 61, 62, 85, 90, 92, 93, 101, 106, 113, 116, 125, 127, 128, 129, 130, 131, 136, 151, 160, 227, 272n.
Intracellular recording, 187
Iproniazid, 194
Irma dream, Freud's, 94–102, 108, 109, 110–11, 119, 124–25, 150, 217, 224–29, 231, 272n.–74n.
Isoniazid, 194–95

Jackson, Hughlings, 2, 9, 161

James, Williams, 133
Janet, Pierre, 75, 79, 86
Jet lag, 37
Johns Hopkins University, 27
Jones, Ernest, 78, 80, 130, 133, 147
Jouvet, Michel, 46, 48, 50, 209
Jung, Carl, 130–33, 137, 139–46, 152, 203, 228, 235, 238, 244

Kandel, Eric, 266n.
Kardiner, Abram, 129–30, 147–49, 157
Kasamatsu, Takaji, 239
Killing bite, 175–77
Kleitman, Nathaniel, 35–37, 40–44, 47, 49–51, 55
Klüver, Heinrich, 32
Klüver-Bucy syndrome, 32
Krafft-Ebing, Richard von, 128
Kubie, Lawrence, 235, 236

Lamarckian inheritance of ideas, 145
Lamella, 185–87, 201, 266n.–67n.
  basic hippocampal circuit within, 196–97, 198, 199
Language, 24–25
  and brain mechanisms for unconscious integration, 217–19
  critical period for acquisition of, 163, 166–69, 178
Lateral geniculate nucleus, 18–19, 23
Learning, 179, 189
  as integrative process, 205, 220
Le Havre, 75
Lenneberg, Eric, 168
Leyhausen, Paul, 174–77, 179, 184, 208, 209
Libet, Benjamin, 234, 276n.–78n., 279n.
Libido theory, 133–36
Lichtheim, Anna Hammerschlag, 272n.–73n.
Limbic system, 60, 186, 190, 239

anatomy of, 29–30, 32–*33*
function of, 31–32, 34, 241–42
and neuronal gating in
    hippocampus, 193–202
Line detection, 169, 170, 172–73
Lithium, 237
Lobotomy, 10, *24*, 195
Locus coeruleus, 193
Long-term memory, 15–17, 213
Lynch, Gary, 266n.

McLean, Paul, 30
Macrides, Foteos, 268n.
Mammals, marsupial and placental,
    204, 206, 241
  sleep cycle in, 53, 56
Mammillary bodies, 30–31, *32–33*
Manic-depressive psychosis, 156
  and physical brain function, 236–
    37
Marie, 79
Marie Bonaparte, Princess, 118,
    272n.
Masochism, 102–3, 136
Masturbation, 232
Mayer, Robert, 145
Memory, 128, 177–78, 179, 207,
    252n.–53n., 279n.
  consolidation of, 212–13, 233, 242
  and dreams, *116*, 212
  and hippocampal interaction with
    neocortex, 201
  and H.M.'s syndrome, 11–17
  and hysteria, 81–85
  and information processing in
    REM sleep, 206–12
  long-term, 15–17, 213
  repression of, 92–93
  See also Amnesia
Mental disorders, 62, 71, 156–57,
    243
  and the limbic system, 34
  and monoamine
    neurotransmitters, 194–95
  physical basis of, 235–40

See also individual conditions
Mesmer, Anton, 76–77
Meyer, Adolf, 133
Meynert, Theodor, 63, 66, 79
Milligan, Billy, 76, 88
Milner, Brenda, 12–13, 17
Mishkin, Mortimer, *24*, 28–29,
    253n.–54n.
Monoamine oxidase, 194
Monoamines, 192–95, 238
Monotremes, 53–*59*, 204–5, 243
Montefiore Hospital, 210
Montreal Neurological Institute, 11–
    12
Morphine, 96, 97, 123
Morrison, Adrian, 46, 209
Moser, Fanny (Frau Emmy von N.),
    79–80, 81
Motor inhibition in REM sleep, 46–
    47, 115, 256n.
Motor output, 31, 58
Mountcastle, Vernon, 27
Mt. Zion Hospital, 234
Movement perception, 24, *25*, 26–
    27
Multiple personality, 6, 68–71, 147
  and hysteria, 74–77, 87, 88
  physical basis of, 235–36
Muzio, Joseph, 51
Myths, 145

Nagel, Ernest, 153
Narcissistic character disorders, 157
National Institute of Mental Health,
    28
National Institutes of Health, 30
Neocortex, 34, *56*, 58, 206
  and alpha rhythm generation, 38–
    39
  anatomy of, *24–25*, 30, *32–33*
  and cortical column
    neuroanatomy, 185, 201, 241–
    42
  critical period in development of,
    162, *163–64*, 178–79

EEG frequencies in, 181–*82*
and hippocampal theta rhythm,
    180, 188, 189, 266n.
and memory consolidation, 213
and neuronal gating in
    hippocampus, 193, 197–202
and sensory perception, 18–*19*,
    24–25, 26–27
and sleep, 35, 43–44
and the unconscious, 219–20
Neo-Freudian psychoanalysts, 139,
    150–51
Neural mechanisms
and critical period in brain
    development, 162–79
and hippocampal theta rhythm,
    180–91
neuronal gating in hippocampus,
    193–202
Neuroleptics, 195
Neurosis, 6, 89, 93, 144, 149, 156–
    57, 221
physical basis of, 235, 245
and unconscious conflicts, 115
Neurotransmitters, *22*, 192–95, 235,
    237
function of, 21
and schizophrenia, 238–40
New Yorker, The, 159
New York Psychoanalytic
    Association, 147
Norepinephrine, 192–95
and mental disorders, 237, 238,
    239
and neural processing in
    hippocampus, 196, 201, 270n.
Nothnagel, Hermann, 66

Obsessional neurosis, 115, 146, 149,
    157
Ocular dominance columns, 169,
    170, 171, 173
Oedipus complex, 105–6, 117, 148–
    49, 153, 154, 155, 156, 227,
    229

Adler's view of, 138–39, 152
Jung's view of, 139, 143–44
neo-Freudian view of, 151
Oral stage, 134

Pain threshold, 37
Papez, James, 31–32, 254n.
Pappenheim, Bertha. *See* Anna O.
Paradoxical sleep, 46
Paralysis, hysterical, 71, 72, 146,
    279n.
Parietal cortex, *25*
Pearlman, Chester, 225
Penfield, Wilder, 11, 13–14
Perception, 166
and emotion, 29, 31–34
and H.M.'s syndrome, 16–17
See also Sensory perception
Personality, 245
Freudian view of, 3–4, 117
neo-Freudian view of, 150
physical basis of, 235, 238
and prefrontal damage, 59
and psychosurgery, 10–11
unconscious, 228–29, 244
Peterfreund, Emanuel, 155
Pettigrew, John, 239
Phenothiazines, 195
Philosophy, 144
Phobias, 106, 146, 157
Phonemic perception, 163, 166–69,
    178–79
"Physical Mechanisms of Hysterical
    Phenomena, On the," 87
Piaget, Jean, 279n.
Pleasure principle, 134
Popper, Karl, 153
Postsynaptic membrane, *22*
Preconscious, 114, *116*, 135, 233,
    234, 235, 276n.
and psychoanalytic goal, 117
Predation, 207, 208
critical period in, 162, 174–79
and sleep cycle evolution, 53
and theta rhythm, 183–84

Prefrontal cortex, 24–25, 178, 179, 185, 204
  evolutionary development of, 206–9
  function of, 58–59, 205–6
  of schizophrenics, 238–40
  species variation in, 56–57
  and the unconscious, 219–20
Prefrontal lobotomy, 10, 24
Primary visual cortex, 18–19, 20, 21, 23–25, 27, 28, 239
  and alpha rhythm generation, 38–39
  connections within, 169, 170, 171
  and REM sleep, 43, 46
Primates, 185, 190
Prince, Morton, 75–76, 147
Procedural memory, 16–17
"Project for a Scientific Psychology," 118, 263n.
"Proposed Mechanism of Emotion, A," 31
Psychic energy, 133
Psychoactive drugs, 21, 157, 193–95, 235
Psychoanalysis, 3–6, 94, 111, 220, 243–45
  critics of, 151–56
  current state of, 157–60
  dreams as influenced by, 227
  goal of, 117, 125–26
  history of, 127–47, 150–51
  methods of, 147–50, 158
  origin of, 66–73, 77–90
  as a therapy, 156–57
  and World War I, 146–47
Psycho-history, 263n.
Psychopathia Sexualis, 128
Psychopathology of Everyday Life, The, 128
Psychosis, 157
  physical basis of, 235, 236–40
  and psychosurgery, 10–11, 13
Psychosurgery, 10–11, 13
Punishment dreams, 103, 136
Puns, 112

Pupillary responses, 170
Puységur, Marquis de, 77
Pyramidal cell, 21

Ramon y Cajal, Santiago, 2, 270n.
Ranck, James, Jr., 188
Rapid eye movement (REM) sleep, 103, 243
  biology of, 40–56, 59
  critical period impressions processed during, 220–21
  evolution of, 204, 241
  information processing during, 206–12
  memory activation during, 213
  motor inhibition during, 46–47, 115, 256n.
  and neural processing in hippocampus, 193, 197–98, 200–2
  theta rhythm during, 184–85, 188–90
Reaction formation, 152–53, 154
Rechtschaffen, Allan, 49
Reflex neurosis, 118
Religion, 144–45, 159
REM rebound, 48–49
REM sleep. See Rapid eye movement (REM) sleep
Representability, 108, 112, 114, 151, 214, 215, 217–19, 274n.
Repression, 131, 139, 146, 151–52, 155, 160, 210, 216, 225, 226, 233, 245, 275n.–76n.
  and dreams, 92–93, 103, 114–15, 214
  and the ego, 136
  and hysteria, 81–82, 84
  neo-Freudian view of, 151
  neuropsychological basis for, 234
Reptiles, 55, 189, 204–5, 271n.
Resistance, 139, 275n.
Respiratory rate, 35–36, 41
Retina, 18–19, 22–23

Rie, Oskar, 94, 98, 101, 102, 272n.–73n.
RNA synthesis, 56
Rockefeller University, 232
Roffwarg, Howard, 51–52, 210–12, 220
Role playing, 221
Rush Presbyterian St. Luke's Medical Center, 221

Salk Institute, 193
Salpêtrière, the, 66, 67, 71–75, 77, 78
Scalp electrodes, 187
Schizophrenia, 34, 71, 131, 156
    and the monoamines, 194–95
    and physical brain function, 237–40
Schur, Max, 119, 124–25, 225, 226, 233
Science, 47
Scoville, William, 10–13, 253n.
Secondary elaboration, 114–15, 116
Sensitive period. See Critical period
Sensory cortex, 178, 242
Sensory perception, 4, 58, 186, 190, 207
    brain mechanisms of, 18–29
    critical period for, 162–64, 178–79
    and the norepinephrine system, 193
    See also Hearing; Visual system
Septum, 30, 32–33, 267n.
Serotonin, 192–95, 237, 238
    and neural processing in hippocampus, 196
Sexuality, 100–1, 128, 131
    in dreams, 227, 230–32
    and libido theory, 133–36
    See also Infant sexuality theory
Sexual orientation, 117, 155–56
    See also Homosexuality
Sexual symbolism, 112–15

Sexual trauma, 81, 83–84, 86, 87, 88–89
Sibling rivalry, 104–5, 227
Sleep, 5, 213–14, 243
    biology of, 34–60
    evolutionary history of, 50, 53–60
    and hippocampal theta rhythm, 180
    life span development of, 50–53
    thought processes during, 210–12
    See also Rapid eye movement (REM) sleep; Sleep deprivation; Slow-wave sleep
Sleep deprivation, 37, 47–49, 243
Sleep-onset periods, 210–14
Sleepwalking, 256n.
Slips of the tongue, 128
Slow-wave sleep, 44–45, 187
    evolution of, 55–56
    information processing in, 208, 210
    and neural processing in hippocampus, 193, 197–98, 200–2
Smell, 18, 24, 58, 190
Social class, 74, 79, 157
Societal environment, 235, 246–47
Solloway, Frank, 70
"Some Additional Day Residues of the Specimen Dream of Psychoanalysis," 119
Soul, 159–60
Spatial imagery, 24
Species-specific behaviors, 207–8, 213, 243
    theta rhythm associated with, 183–85, 188–90, 268n.
Species survival, 184, 188, 190, 207
    See also Evolution
Specimen dream. See Irma dream, Freud's
Speech, 2
    in dreams, 112
Sperry, Roger, 232
Spindles, 40
Spinelli, Nico, 173

Spirit, 144–45, 232
Squire, Larry, 14–16, 212
Stanford University, 42, 173
Stekel, Wilhelm, 129, 140
Stoller, Robert, 244
Studies on Hysteria, 81, 87, 88, 128, 131
Subconscious, 233
  See also Preconscious
Suggestibility, 77, 156, 220
Sullivan, Harry Stack, 150
Superego, 103, 135–36, 150, 152, 153
Symbolism in dreams, 230, 232
  as expressive means, 214–17
  as repressed material, 108, 112–15, 146, 151, 216
Synapse, 19
Synaptic cleft, 21, *22,* 194
Synaptic facilitation, 178–79, 266n.

Taste, 18, *24*
Thalamus, 18–*19,* 26, 58, 205, 242
Theta rhythm, hippocampal, 7, 46, 191, 196, 207, 208, 266n.–67n.
  and arousal state, 181–83
  function of, 189–90
  and hippocampal structure, 185–86
  neurophysiological mechanisms responsible for, 186–89
  species-specific behaviors associated with, 183–85, 188–90, 268n.
Three Essays on the Theory of Sexuality, 128, 133
Three Faces of Eve, The, 76, 88
Touch, 18, *24–25,* 27, 29
Traité de l'Hystérie, 73
Tranquilizers, 195
Transference, 139, 150, 154, 155, 158, 160, 210, 225, 227, 234
  identified by Freud, 135
  neo-Freudian view of, 151
Traumatic hysteria, 71–72

Traumatic neuroses, 134–35, 147
Tricyclic antidepressants, 194

Unconscious, 139, 160, 244
  brain mechanisms underlying, 34, 204–39, 245, 279n.
  and the critical period, 179, 220–21
  current view of, 151
  and dreams, 111, 114, *116,* 214–19, 241
  Freud's view of, 3–5, 7, 85, 105, 111, 114, *116,* 118, 133, 135, 214, 275n.
  Jung's view of, 131, 144–46, 228
  and REM sleep function, 209–12
  and repression, 92–93, 103–4, 114, 279n.
Unconscious personality, 228–29, 244
University of California at Irvine, 266n.
University of California at Los Angeles, 59, 180
University of California at San Diego, 14
University of California at Santa Cruz, 216
University of Cambridge, 172
University of Chicago, 32, 35, 49
University of Colorado, 49
University of Lund, 238
University of Lyons, 46
University of Pennsylvania, 46
University of Vienna, 63, 128

Vienna Psychoanalytic Society, 129, 130
Violence, 246–47
Visual system, 18–29, 71
  critical period in, 162, 169–74, 178–79
Vogel, Gerald, 49

von N., Emmy (Fanny Moser), 79–80, 81
von R., Elisabeth, 80, 81

War neuroses, 134–35, 146–47, 279n.–80n.
Weil, Dr., 123, 124
Wiesel, Torsten, 22, 169, 170, 171
Wish fulfillment theory, 86, 94–98, 135–36, 146, 152, 222, 223, 224

inadequacy of, 155
Wit and Its Relation to the Unconscious, 128
Women, 73–74, 81
Word association tests, 131, 152
Word perception, 168
Words in dreams, 112
Working through, 149–50
Wundt, Wilhelm, 131

Yale University, 53, 220